Placenta

the Forgotten Chakra

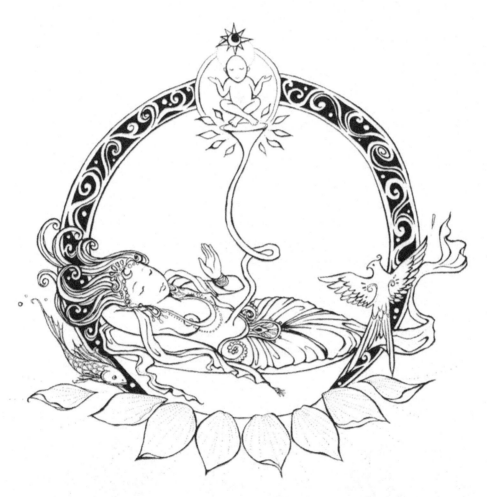

by Robin Lim

illustrated by Miyuki Akiyama

Half Angel Press
P.O. Box 116, Ubud
Bali, Indonesia - 80571

Illustrations by Miyuki Akiyama
Cover design by Zion Lee
Book design by Lakota Moira
Edited by Devin Bramhall, Wil Hemmerle

Photograph on page 27, 37, 40, 147 by Margo Berdeshevsky
Photograph on page 178 by Leon Vrielink
Photograph on page iv, 74, by Luciana Ferrero
Photograph on page 16, 44, 45, 47, 60 by Wil Hemmerle
Photograph on page 93, 118 by Déjà Bernhardt
Photograph on page 84, 96 by Elena Skoko
Photograph on page 129 by Loren Earle-Cruickshanks
Other photos from Bumi Sehat archives

Illustrations on page 11, 67, 126 by Gede Robi
Illustrations on page viii, 46 by Sophia Anastasia
Printed in Bali, Indonesia

This edition ISBN: 0-9762907-7-4

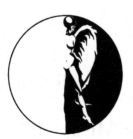 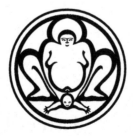 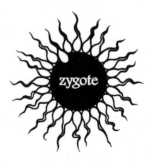

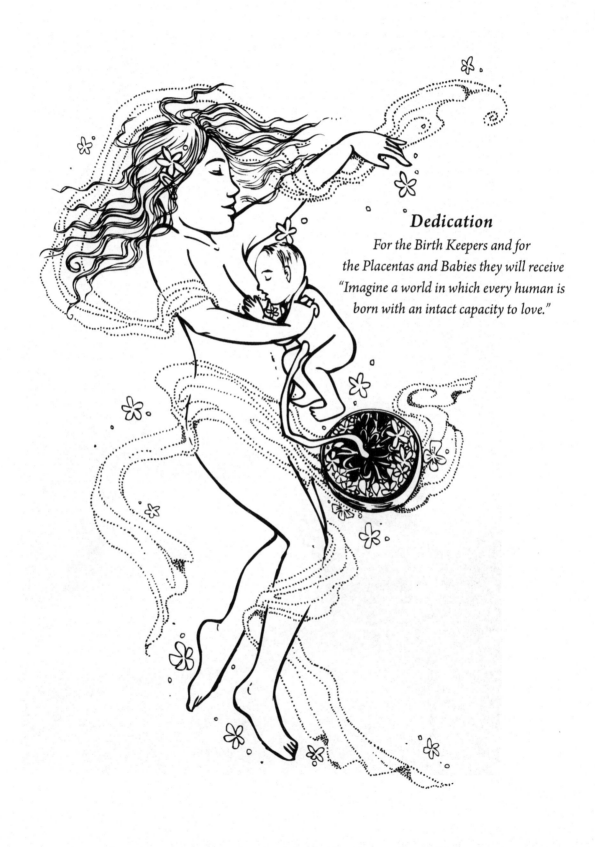

Dedication

For the Birth Keepers and for
the Placentas and Babies they will receive
"Imagine a world in which every human is
born with an intact capacity to love."

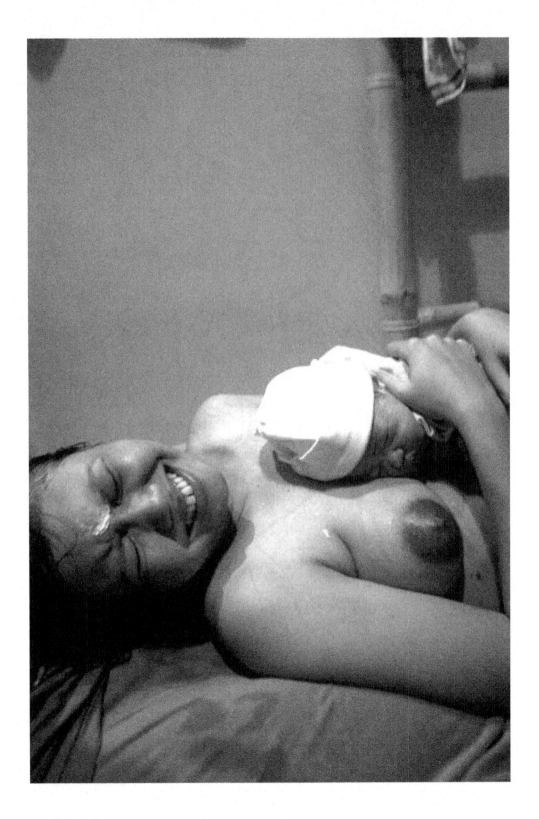

iv

Table of Contents

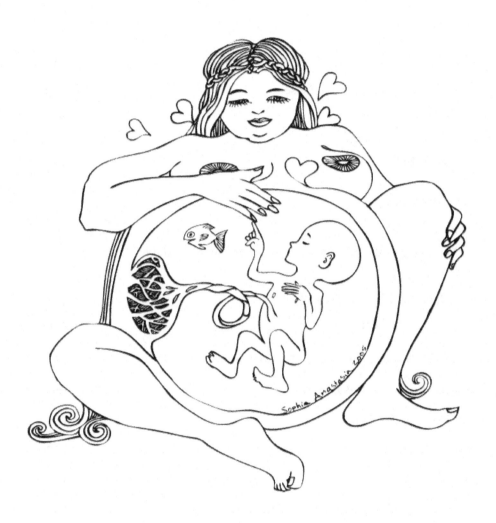

Acknowledgments

It takes a special patience to live with a woman who is in love with placentas, Mothers and Babies. For support, understanding, and for music I thank my husband, Wil Hemmerle. My inspiration has ever been my children, Déjà, Noël, Zhòu, Lakota, Zion, Thoreau, Hanoman and EllyAnna. Hugs for my son-in-love, Robi, daughter-in-love, Edwine, and grandchildren, Zhouie, Bodhi and Tashi. To my mom, Cresencia Munar Lim Jehle and my Lola the healer and baby catcher, Hilot, Vicenta Munar Lim, I owe everything.

Artist Miyuki Akiyama you have blessed these pages. Cover artist, Zion Lee, additional art by Sophia Anastasia. Photographers, Leon Vrielink, Margo Berdeshevsky, Déjà Bernhardt, plus Bumi Archives. Thank you. Copy editors, Wil Hemmerle and Devin Bramhall, you even hemorrhaged for this book. Thank you for a beautiful book design, Lakota Moira of Akarumput, your devotion makes me cry.

Rodney and Team 1st World Library, to have this, a real book in people's hands, is a dream come true. Bruce Grady, you surely are the Midwife of the hardcopy of the English edition of this book!

Team Yayasan Bumi Sehat Bali & International (Healthy Mother Earth Foundation) you are the people who prove it's possible to build world peace, one MotherBaby at a time. The Gentle Birth Midwives/Bidans; Jero Susanti, Brenda Ritchmond, AA Sayang, Ni Ketut Suastini, Dewa Rutini, AA Mas, Ni Made Suastini, Wayan Surdarni, Katherine Bramhall CPM, Maria Marat, Budi Astuti, Yeshi Aprillia S.Si.T M. Kes., Erin Ryan CPM, Lianne Schwartz, Carly Facius

Team Bumi Sehat in Aceh Tsunami Relief Clinic; Dr. Eman Tuahta, Mimi and Leman Wijaya, Midwives: Louise Noorbergen, Nursiyah, Mega Purba, Lisa Forasacco, Maria dalle Pezze, Ibu Cheryl. Love and a deep healing breath to Kelly Dunn, Rene Bisnaire and all the volunteers, staff and supporters of Bumi Sehat Haiti, 2010.

A very huge hug for the Bumi Wadah Medical Relief and Childbirth Camp Team, together we responded to the Typhoon Haiyan Disaster in the Philippines, and have proven that delaying the clamping and cutting of Babies' umbilical cords is essential for survival, especially in the lowest resource/highest risk places on Earth. Maraming Salamat: Teresa Maniego, Lucibelle Kyamko, Toba Pearl, Tina Ferreros, Alfredo Torno III, Jun Ferreros, Marriam, Maita Manglapus, midwives, medics, nurses and doctors : Lorina Solis, Maria Theresa Palaña, Joana Maria Abrenio, Jill Roxanne Montejo, Rhodora Caidic, Maria Filomena Neri, Myra Briones, Lillian

Sanpere Tarragona, Claudia Booker, Vicki Penwell, Rose Penwell, Ian Penwell, Lyn Stark, Jacquelyn Aurora, Celina Szwinta, Dr. Nikko Peven-Izu, Dr. Marissa Casals, Michelle Buenaventura, Karen Ferreira, Sora Colvin, Dr. Valerie Simonsen, Kelly Milligan, Diane Albright, Heather Sadiechild Harris, Susan Holland, Katherine Sims, Claire Jackson, Nienke de Leeuw, Erika & Dillon Carpenter. Our support team; Belly Cañada, Garry Guevarra, Joel Bartolome, Je-ar Ambrona, Nida Ligo, Emma Bell. Ibu Anie Djojohadikusumo, Wadah Foundation Family and Direct Relief International.

Other medical professionals, true healers I have had the pleasure of working with: Dr. Bobbi Aqua DOC, Dr. I Nyoman Hariyasa Sanjaya, SpOG, Dr. Dewa Ketut Arika Seputra, SpOG, Dr. Made Wedagama SpOG, Dr. John Briley MD pediatrics, Dr. Ni Gusti Ayu Partiwi Surjadi, SpA. MARS, Mangku Ketut Liyar, Niccolo Giovannini OBGYN.

Thank you to the Sakthi Foundation: Pradheep, Priya & Panav Chhalliyil and Bruce Grady. Groups who have supported my journey and the work of Bumi Sehat include: Ikatan Bidan Indonesia (IBI), North American Registry of Midwives (NARM), IMAP Integrated Midwives association of the Philippines, Gentle Birth in the Philippines, World Alliance for Breastfeeding Action (WABA), DONA, La Leche league Int., Genius in Diapers, Midwives Alliance of North America (MANA), Delayed Cord Clamping uk, and Hygieia College.

Birth~Keepers & Peace~Keepers who have inspired me include: Marie Zenack & Family, Devin Bramhall, Paula Baudoux, Katia, Margo Berdeshevsky, Gina Maria Catena, Liz Gilbert, Carla Swanson, Michael Franti & Sara, Mala Light, Barbara McLeod Montani, Shawna Wentz, Robbie Davis-Floyd, Ina May Gaskin, Agnes Gereb, Devi Lestari, Reza Gunawan, Ibu Oppie Andaresta, Kurt & kai, George M. Morley, Wallaby Pulsatilla, Farfalla Vitalba, Stefanie Dawn, Julie Gerland, Faye Read, Ronnie Falcao, Gloria Lemay, Rebecca Bashara, Scott, Surreal & Inti, Mark, Gabriel & Aurea Ament, Chiaki, Gerry, Chiyo & Liang Ong, Lya, Diego & Ara, Ratna, Hajis & daughters, Oma Frederika Nault, Sara Wickham, Dr. Sarah J. Buckley , Deb Puterbaugh, Sera Bonds, Rosie Estrin, Viktor Tichy, Uta Meiner, Marianne Littlejohn, Jeanice Barcelo, Orango Riso, Michel Odent, Rico & Clair Baker, Robyn Garrison, Debby Lowry, Mary Jackson, Tina Garzero, Kadi Mourningstar, Jan Francisco, Joanne Dugas, Anne Frye, Nancy Wainer, Marcy Tardio, Nan Koehler, Pearl Breitbach, Diane Frank, Faith Gibson, Kate Bowland, Roxanne Potter, Mary Offerman, Lance Sims, Melody Weig, Beverly Francis, Rahima Baldwin, Valerie El Halta, Raven Lang, Lori Land, Elizabeth Davis, Kalanete, Marina, Joseph Yacoe & children, Marjan deJong, Pamela Hunt, Hannelore Josam, Ni Ketut Rusni, Sam,

Prajna & Zion Shapiro, Marietta Paragas, Gina Tyler, Alesia Lloyd, Linda & Babu Walling, Andy Carmone, Suzanne Arms, Jan Tritten, Ida Daragh, Ashisha and Peggy O'Mara, Sandra Morningstar, Lee & Chris Beckom, Elena Skoko, Rob Bluebird & Koko, Stacy, "the Girls" & Andy Gunter, each of you has helped tremendously because you have believed in our vision.

Giuditta Torenetta, Debra Pascali-Bonaro, Marzia Bisognin, Chiara Pozzi Perteghella, Roberta Plevani, and all the Doulas who Mother the Mothers. Thank you. Dr. Eden Gabrielle Fromberg, a hug.

Special blessings rain down on me from the BirthKeepers who have passed over; Sunny Supplee, Mary Kroeger, Jeannine Parvati, June Whitson, Stephen Gaskin, Sharon Evans, Marsden Wagner, Carolyn Sims, Kerry Pendergast, Cristina Abbio, Gina Sitz, Ibu Rindi, Theodore Sturgeon, Wayan Budiyasa, Zoe Christian, Dawn Teddi Wiedemann, Christine Jehle Kim and my father, Robert A. Jehle.

Thank you APPPAH Association for Pre-and Perinatal Psychology and Health, for giving me the honor of BirthKeeper of the Year, in the gentle lap of Jeannine Parvati, who first opened my heart to loving placentas as well as MotherBaby. Most profoundly I thank the Alexander Langer Foundation for giving me the opportunity to walk in the footsteps Alex Langer, a pilgrim for peace on Earth. Friends & Family in Italy: Maurizio Rosenberg Colorni, Sabina Langer, Anastasia Mostacci, Marzia Bisognin. Much love to, Verena Schmid, Valentina Facchin, Lisa Forasacco, Maria dalle Pezze, Gloriana Facci and the wonderful Bianca Buchal, Il Melograno Natural Childbirth centers throughout Italy, especially Tiziana Valpiana, Grazie!

Everyone in every country who voted for me for CNN Hero… you gave your hearts to build a platform for Gentle Childbirth to become stronger. Dear parents of the future, go gently with the babies they are a collection of our passions, keep them intact, and breastfeed, please. Gentle Birth families, thank you for the courage to reinvent humanity, This is how we build peace. I love you all so much.

Preface

This book grapples with the miracle of sexual reproduction, with all its complexities. Would it be possible to speak of mothers, babies or their placentas without delving into the realm of Spirit? Of course not, sexuality is sacred territory. Yet for me, the concept of religion/spirituality is a complete mystery. I don't have a clue what "God" or "God-us" must or could look like. I would like to have the ability to name what it is exactly I believe in, but I cannot. I have no answers for my spiritual questions, and no name for the benevolence that I pray exists. This not a comfortable place to be, but for me it is honest. And so, this book begins here, with my indescribable, and perhaps unanswerable questions: "What is the meaning of our birth?" "Are we, each of us, a piece of peace?" "Where does spirit live inside of us?" "Was it in our placentas, which is why most of us feel we've lost something meaningful and essential?" I have the courage to hope that the discussion I begin here, and share with each of you, will revolutionize birth.

My dear friend and 'sister witch' told me she dreamed the universe was writing a book, and making me do the work. This is that book, Marie. Thank you for dreaming.

Feeling all this, and writing about it, gives me immense faith that we stand on the cusp of such possibility, to begin gently greeting optimal humans into this world. I believe in a benevolent hand that dreams this universe into existence. This hand moves for me when I trust in utter uncertainty. As a midwife, this is the humble place, the center from which I must work. For I have experienced that whatever I need, to do the service I do for my mothers and babies, is always at my fingertips. If I think I need something and it is not available, it turns out that something better, more suitable, is just in front of my eyes. I only need pay attention, and be open to that still small voice of guidance and inspiration. Even if that voice is telling me to do something very strange compared to what is considered normal midwifery protocol, like leave the umbilical cord, baby and placenta intact! Or perhaps, write a book all about placentas.

Introduction

The placenta, the root of your origin, is a miraculous organ that shares and protects your life. It is the conductor that unites you with your mother and serves as the control panel of the womb-ship that sustains you until you are born. It was conceived at the moment of your genesis. Your placenta is genetically identical to you. Though you share some of your parents' genetic identity, unless you have a monozygotic (identical) twin, no one, except your placenta, has ever been so perfectly, exactly you. Sexual reproduction, the act of creating new life, only works because of the placenta. As mammals, we reproduce sexually, so sex is the reddest, hottest tile in the mosaic of our earthly lives, and the placenta is the mandala in the center of this miracle. Historically, our creation stories tell of the Earth Mother birthing the world: her amniotic fluid became the oceans, the placenta became the Tree of Life. This demonstrates how essential the placenta is to our survival and how embedded it is in our psyche.

According to Chaos Theory, dynamic systems are sensitive to start up conditions. Human beings are extremely dynamic systems, and our survival hinges on the strength of our individual immune systems. The placenta is the commander-in-chief of the baby's immune system during embryonic development (i.e. condition of start-up). Thus, we must protect our offspring's placentas by being gentle during the transition of birth, to give our children the best possible start and protect the very foundation of their immune systems.

Epigenetics (the study of inherited changes in gene expression caused by something other than DNA) is opening our minds to the understanding that the way genes express themselves is more complicated than simply adding together the genetic contributions encoded in mother and father. What mother eats, drinks, feels and experiences in her environment has an impact on the offspring's future health intelligence and entire genetic manifestation. All of this impacts the gestating child and will radiate out to her future generations. The conduit between mother's gestalt of experiences is the umbilical cord and the placenta is the organ of synthesis. Is it any wonder that placentas have been considered angels in many traditions?

Look down at your navel. There is undoubtedly a small depression or scar left by the detachment of your umbilical cord, right at the center of your body. This is a permanent mark, a souvenir reminder of your placenta, which was crucial to your development as an embryo and fetus. Yet, in our modern culture, we do not think about our umbilical cords and placentas. Most hospitals in the west today simply dispose of the babies' placentas, tossing them out as mere medical waste. How did the placenta, central to our survival and future well-being, lose its significance and come to be considered garbage? This was born of an ugly revolution in the twentieth century and driven by society's momentum to dominate nature, which Dr. Michel Odent, who specializes in Obstetrics and helped popularize water birth, calls "the industrialization of childbirth."

The natural process of bringing new human life into the world became a medical event in which the mother-to-be was hospitalized, drugged and the baby was delivered from her, not by her. Somehow in an attempt to make childbirth safe, science was employed preemptively, and birth became a highly technological rushed process of rescuing the baby from the womb. For babies the transition into earthly life became a harsh succession of protocols in which the mother's perineum was cut to widen the vagina and speed up the birth. The baby, often unresponsive due to drugs given to the mother during labor, was handled roughly, even hung upside down and spanked to stimulate breathing. The umbilical cord was immediately clamped and cut with no attention paid to the long-term trauma caused by jarring discordant separation of baby from mother and placenta. Mother was taken to a recovery room to rest, while the baby she had carried under her heart for nine months was isolated in a box and fed from a bottle. Placenta, the heroine of gestation, was tossed in the rubbish for incineration. The miracle, which once belonged to families, was now the property of medical establishments. Medical science, which, when applied wisely saved lives, lost its way in the territory of childbirth. Medicine became divorced from nature and forgot to respect the diversity of human culture and tradition. Somehow in the application of such efficiency, we lost our humanity at the fulcrum of the most tender of life's moments: the birth of a child.

At birth, it is important to be sure that the baby, placenta, mother and family are truly ready for the umbilical cord to be cut. This first cut irrevocably severs the physical bond between baby and his or her placental angel. In addition, birth-keepers, I believe that if the cord is to be severed at all, it is important to do this with reverence and pure intention, since once the baby-cord-placenta trinity is broken, it cannot be restored. Ask the placenta and the baby, "Is this OK with you?" Say a silent prayer, asking forgiveness for the separation caused by the severance of the cord. Take your time! Go slowly! There is no need to hurry or worry. Remember: cutting the cord is not a rescue operation, though to see it done it hospitals you would think it is. It is indeed the rushing and the cutting that we need to rescue babies from.

Philosophers of every age have wondered where the seat of the Soul is. Is it in the body's brain or in the heart? Some cultures have postulated that the eternal human soul lives in the liver or kidneys. My observation has been this: Since our conception we each shared the womb with our placenta. Your placenta grew with you. During gestation your placenta protected you and your mother, bringing essential nutrients and oxygen and removing waste via the labyrinth of placental circulation and the separate but cooperating pathways of your mother's blood stream. So, my question is: Do our placentas also have souls? Or, do we share our soul with our placentas?

This book is an exploration, born of my fascination, respect and even love for placentas. I believe in asking questions, even if the answers may never be fulfilled, it is the question that provides the spiritual pathway to astonishment. If you are reading this, you too must have an interest in your intricate spiritual roots and human inception. Welcome to a storybook, about your placenta, the Tree of Life, the source, the forgotten Chakra. Here light will be shed on the placenta's functions: physiologically, historically and culturally. If we think of a human life as a lotus plant: the placenta is the root, the cord is the stem and the baby the flower/fruit, perhaps, by watering this root in our hearts, some sense can be made of our lives. By nurturing where we come from, we may find clues as to where we are going. On this ailing planet, in our troubled times, may we embrace our origins and nourish our potential, to light our way safely home.

For this book, I have chosen to use she/her pronouns. It is not a sign of preferential treatment, but I had to choose. In Bali, the male babies are valued much higher than female. Here I wish only to establish a balance.

"Late clamping (or not clamping at all) is the physiological way of treating the cord, and early clamping is an intervention that needs justification. The "transfusion" of blood from the placenta to the infant, if the cord is clamped late, is physiological, and adverse effects of this transfusion are improbable...

...but in normal birth there should be a valid reason to interfere with the natural procedure." [1]

– World Health Organization

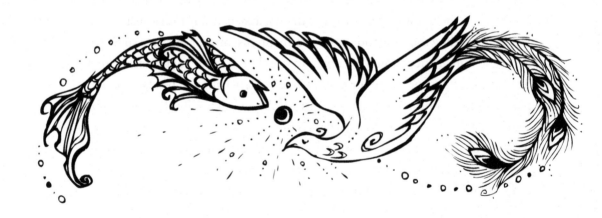

What is the Placenta?

Fertilization: the miracle that occurs when the sperm meets the egg after two people make love. Imagine the 500 to 700 million sperm cells from the father's ejaculation hurtling toward one glistening egg inside the mother. It is the first marathon of a new life. The winner, the most fit, arrives at the right moment and is allowed by the egg to enter. Together they unite and become a zygote, the first cell of a new human. The first day after fertilization of the ovum, the unity begins to diversify: first cleavage and division, now there are two cells, then quickly four, and by day three of gestation eight cells called blastomeres have evolved. These then multiply into sixteen cells called morula, and the process continues.

Seed of Life

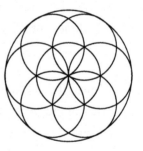

Quickly after conception four cells are created. By day three they have multiplied into eight cells called blastomeres and day four, sixteen cells are achieved called the morula.

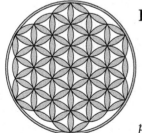

Flower of Life

As our embryo begins it's second week of life the 3 to 4 day process of implantation transpires and is normally complete by day 12. The amniotic sac develops and cradles the embryo as outgrowths of the trophoblast project into the endometrium (lining of the uterus) and become the placenta, the mandala or flower of life, well planted. This is what I call the sacred geometry of splitting souls.

During this rapid growth the entire package is traveling down the fallopian tube toward the uterine cavity, a welcoming bed-womb complete with room service. By day five after fertilization, implantation is initiated, trophoblast cells, a layer of tissue on the outside of the blastula, begin to form the placenta and the inner cell mass of the blastocyst differentiate to become the body of the baby. Placenta and baby spring from the union of sperm and egg, and their shared origin reveals them as genetically identical.

Day six after fertilization the trophoblast cells of the placenta begin to attach to the inside of the uterine wall. As the embryo begins its second week of life, implantation continues to transpire and is typically complete by day twelve. Next, the amniotic sac develops to cradle the embryo while outgrowths of the trophoblast project into the endometrium (lining of the uterus) and form the placenta. By now, the developing placenta has completely embedded itself inside the mother's uterus. Placental circulation and maternal circulation begin to make exchanges, yet the mother's blood does not enter or mix with the infantile placenta. From the beginning of the third month of the pregnancy the fetus and the mother maintain completely separate blood systems. This is one of the miracles of the placenta: it both integrates mother and child while also maintaining their integrity as individual and separate systems. For example, nutrients and oxygen diffuse from maternal blood into fetal blood, yet, amazingly, baby and mother sometimes maintain different blood types.

The umbilical cord is composed of one vein that carries oxygenated, nutrient-rich blood to the fetus, and two arteries that carry deoxygenated, depleted blood from the baby to the mother for her excretory system to dispose of. It is covered with Wharton's jelly, made of mucopolysaccharides. The cord is usually about 50 centimeters long and 2 centimeters in diameter. It is strong and flexible. It ensures a steady supply of enzymes for metabolism, ions of calcium to build bone, and iron to produce blood. Sometimes the umbilical cord has one vein and only one artery, which may be related to fetal abnormalities or may occur without any problems for baby.

The baby also receives oxygen via spiral arteries in the deciduas (thick layer of modified mucous membrane living in the uterine endometrial). The maternal blood flow, under pressure, enters the intervilbus space via the spiral arteries and bathes the placental villi in oxygen-rich blood. Within the placental villi, gasses are exchanged and the maternal blood flow decreases with deoxygenated blood. Total waste products of carbon dioxide flow back via the mother's endometrial veins. Mother's blood and baby's blood in the placenta come close enough to exchange gases, but do not intermingle.

The placenta chooses and transports nutrients needed for the formation of the baby's tissues. It selects these elements from the mother's blood, uses what is necessary and sends it into the blood of the fetus. As a midwife, I have observed over the years that the placenta will try to advocate for the developing baby when the mother is deficient in essential nutrients. For example, malnourished mothers may deliver healthy babies of normal birth weight, while suffering themselves from obvious signs of hunger. Additionally, in the instance of IUFGR (intra-uterine fetal growth restriction) the fetus can use the placenta to signal to the mother that she is in need of more nutrients.[1]

A study in 2001 by Langley-Evens et. al. using rats showed that maternal protein restriction decreased birth weight and placental 11ß-HSD2 activity. The study proposed that maternal undernutrition results in fetal glucocorticoid exposure, which leads to the programming of hypertension in later life. Further work demonstrated that a low protein maternal diet reduced 11ß-HSD2 gene expression in the rat placenta and in the fetal and neonatal kidney and adrenal. The authors suggested that altered exposure of the fetus and, in particular, the fetal kidney to glucocorticoids may lead to the observed increase in GR protein and mRNA expression in the kidney, which was a possible mechanism for raised blood pressure in later life.[2]

This beautiful organ weighs only about one pound and looks very much like a purple, blue and red tree of life (As a world religions major in junior college I became enamored with the concept of a tree of life, its many branches illustrating to me the interrelationships between religious belief, scientific research, philosophy and mythology. In the branches and in the roots I became convinced that all of life is a finely woven web of connections). On the baby's side the placenta is smooth and glossy, the umbilical cord with its two arteries and one vein is attached and radiates outward. On the mother's side the placenta appears more like meat, with a spongy surface that attaches to the interior wall of the uterus. Following parturition (birth) the placenta falls neatly away from the shrinking uterine wall and is born approximately eleven to twenty minutes after the baby. The birth of the placenta is best accomplished without complications if the mother is properly nourished and has the energy reserves necessary to accomplish this third stage of labor.

"The placenta is our second mother. It is Mother Nature nurturing us with her perfection" – Marjan de Jong, a mother in Holland

During pregnancy and after birth, the placenta makes maternal and child survival possible. It provides for our nutritional needs and aids in our development. It acts as a barrier guarding us against harmful bacteria and most foreign molecules. As an organ of synthesis, it manufactures and employs estrogen, progesterone and gonadotropin to keep the mother and baby alive and well from the embryonic period to birth. Progesterone is sometimes called the hormone of pregnancy[3], as it supports gestation and embryogenesis.

Pomegranate, called il melograno in Italy, delima in Indonesia, granada in Spanish, grenadier in French, meyve nar in Turkish, is a beautiful anti-oxidant fruit, found all over the world. With its luscious red color and plump juicy seed filled body, it is a widely accepted symbol of women's fertility. The pomegranate is believed to have power over evil. It is sacred to the Goddesses Persephone, Venus and Inanna. I propose it looks very much like our dear placenta!

When miscarriages happen in the time between conception and placental implantation, it can be due to insufficient progesterone. As the placenta develops and makes it's rich cocktail of hormones, a normal, healthy pregnancy is typically maintained. The placenta secretes hormones that regulate uterine contractions, making the uterus a comfortable cocoon in which the baby can develop. These hormones also prepare the mother's body to lactate, which will be the baby's source of life post partum. Thus, the placenta serves as a crucial life resource for the baby both within the womb and after birth.

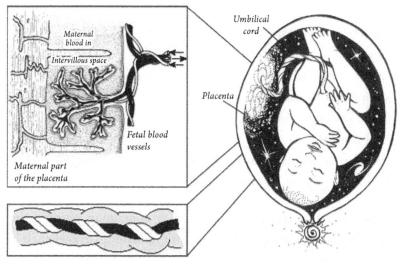

The placenta. The fetal (umbilical) arteries and their branches are shown white, and the vein and its branches black.

"It must not be forgotten that it is the placenta, an organ composed of cells, that is performing the choosing, giving/taking, storing and carrying. For example, it knows when there is a need for iron, chooses the element iron from among other substances and knows how it should be used. It is not a human being that has this knowledge, but a collection of cells called the placenta. The fact that a cell can recognize an element is surely a miracle. What is even more miraculous is that it can take the appropriate material in the required amount and carry it to a particular location. The events that occur in the miracle of human and all mammalian creation indicate a consciousness displayed by the cells, and by the molecules and atoms that produce the cells. Indeed, this consciousness does not belong to any of them, but to God who creates them and inspires in them the functions that they are to perform." [4] – Harun Yahya

The Placenta's Talent for Cloaking

Gestational immune tolerance is simply the absence of the pregnant mom's immune response against the developing baby and placenta. Because the baby is genetically different from the mother, non-rejection is accomplished by a special barrier or privilege between the mother and fetus. The placenta makes this possible on the cellular level, as explained in the book, *Maternal-Fetal Medicine*:

> *"The placental trophoblast cells do not express the classical MHC class I isotypes HLA-A and HLA-B, unlike most other cells in the body, and this absence is assumed to prevent destruction by maternal cytotoxic T cells, which otherwise would recognize the fetal HLA-A and HLA-B molecules as foreign. On the other hand, they do express the atypical MHC class I isotypes HLA-E and HLA-G, which is assumed to prevent destruction by maternal NK cells, which otherwise destruct cells that do not express any MHC class I. However, trophoblast cells do express the rather typical HLA-C."*[5]

In addition, placentas secrete Neurokinin B containing phosphocholine molecules. This is the strategy used by parasitic nematodes to keep their host's immune systems from detecting their presence.

Another strategy used by the placentas of mammals to prevent their mother's from miscarrying them, is to form a syncytium or multi-nucleated interface. This barrier limits the movement of certain kinds of cells between the developing baby and the mother. This syncytial epithelium (interface of special blood cells which are able to insert themselves between epithelial cells) is why the mother's circulation does not mix with the embryo's circulation. Even more miraculous is the fact that while providing this barrier the placenta still allows the mother's antibodies to pass to the fetus, protecting the baby from infection, while not attacking the baby.

In some cases, the placenta maintains the baby's life even after both baby and placenta are born. The first time I experienced this was when our family dog Madu, a mix basset hound, birthed nine puppies. One was stillborn.

Madu licked her stillborn puppy and, even more interesting, she aggressively licked the placenta of the stillborn which was still attached to the pup via the umbilical cord.

I had just read in an article from India that the old Ayurvedic method of reviving the stillborn child was to warm the placenta. Warming the placenta is consistent with the Ayurvedic beliefs about the significance of the placenta. For centuries, the practice of stimulating the placenta if a baby does not breathe or appears lifeless at birth has been practiced in India, Bangladesh and Burma. Warming the placenta with heat (i.e. hot water) or manual stimulation (massage) activates the jeeva (praan or life force) of the child that is stored in the placenta and is passed gradually into the baby after the birth.

I recalled this as I watched Madu continue to lick her pup's placenta, the pup now nestled under Madu's chin. After continuing this for some time, Madu picked up her chin to reveal, miraculously, a living puppy! Madu ate all her pup's placentas, though she did not begin right away. She waited until all nine had been born and the stillborn pup revived. This was an all day process, from dawn into the night. Once she had revived her pup, Madu chose the biggest, strongest pup and ate his placenta. Then she ate the placenta of the next strongest pup. She continued to eat the placentas in that order, until lastly she ate the runt's placenta. Somehow she knew to leave the placenta of the weakest pup attached the longest, thus allowing time for the life force to pass fully from the placenta to the pup.

A few nights later at the Bumi Sehat Birth Center in Bali, I received a stillborn baby into the world. We had never seen her malnourished mother before that night. She began pushing very shortly after she arrived. The baby's heart rate skyrocketed just as she was crowning him and then stopped. The baby was born and did not begin to breathe. His heartbeat was absent and his muscle tone was limp. We immediately began performing CPR while administering oxygen, to no avail. There was no sign of life, yet death did not feel close. Thirteen minutes later, when the placenta was born, I asked the nurse to quickly bring me a bowl of hot water. We placed the placenta, still connected by it's cord to the baby, into the warm water, the baby's grandfather added

Tirtha, holy water from the family temple, and, instantly, the baby shuddered and took a breath. The baby is perfectly healthy and his name is Tirtha.

In India, the "Jeeva Project" proposes investigating the indigenous practice by Dais, traditional birth attendants, of reviving the stillborn or compromised newborn by warming the placenta. At Bumi Sehat birth center in Bali we have found this a very successful method for preserving newborn life. But it only works if the cord is not clamped and/or cut. Since life is still being transferred from placenta to baby after birth, immediate clamping and cutting of the cord sabotages the transference of this life force, so essential for optimal health and well-being.[6]

> The Matrika project recorded placental stimulation from locations in Bihar, Delhi, Rajasthan and Himachal Pradesh (Matrika 2004). A three continent WHO sponsored review of traditional childbirth practices (Lefeber and Voorhoeve 1998) notes that, in case a newborn does not cry after birth, indigenous midwives in Bangladesh, Burma and India heat the placenta and "milk" the cord, and attributes "trampling on the placenta" to Bangladesh. From countries, as far apart as Ghana and Bangladesh, Ethiopia and the Philippines, the same authors point out "practices based on the transfer of life and strength to the baby through the placenta, umbilical cord and anterior fontanelle", and state that "the techniques employed to resuscitate a newborn child demonstrate clearly that the placenta is the seat of some life-matter".[7]

Igarot tribal peoples of the Cordilleria mountains in the Philippine islands hang the placenta high in the trees, so the child will be a free soaring spirit. Many Filipino mothers bury the baby's placenta with a book to insure the child will be intelligent.

What are the Chakras?

chakra |ˈCHäkrə|
noun
(in Indian thought) each of the centers of spiritual power in the
human body, usually considered to be seven in number.
ORIGIN from Sanskrit cakra 'wheel or circle,' from an Indo-
European base meaning 'turn,' shared by wheel.

When it comes to our energy centers, also known as our chakras,
my belief is tempered with pragmatism (imagine a woman who
writes an entire book on placenta saying that she is a pragmatist!). Yet
here I go, jumping into the question: What are the chakras?

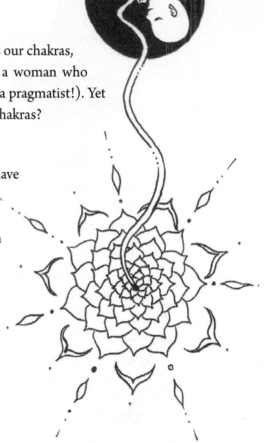

I cannot pretend to understand the mystery of the
chakras fully, but in my research and exploration, I have
come to believe that our chakras are *mandalas* of
energy and light. And this light is what activates our
eternal souls to dwell in our bodies. Human wisdom
from many cultures scattered over our earth and
throughout our history seem to agree:
Our bodies "glow" with centers of spiritual energy
or light or vibration. Many cultures assign each
body-spirit center with specific colors, forming
a rainbow bridge between spiritual energy and the
physical manifestation of life.

Our bodies are conduits for energy, the energy of the soul as it occupies and animates the body. This energy has been described as spiritual, ethereal, magical and even transcendental. My observation is that this indescribable energy, which is like an engine that enlivens and drives the whole body, is focused in certain centers. These energy centers are the chakras. Like a turbine engine, the chakras are wheels that turn as they generate and burn energy.

It is also my observation that these energy centers are beehives of hormonal activity. Being a midwife, I have tremendous respect for the power and delicacy of hormones. The chakra centers of our body, where the power of our soul or spirit energy is most focused, corresponds to the places where our hormones are most concentrated, our endocrine glands (glands that secrete hormones or other products directly into the blood). Perhaps this very fact is the reason that most all of our world's religions guide us to be balanced. Even a slight imbalance in our hormones can be profoundly uncomfortable, both spiritually and physically. It is the hormones which seem to be the bridge between our physical bodies and the spirit energy of our souls.

Each one of us is a soul possessing a body. Sadly, in our hyper-materialistic world many of us become unconsciously convinced that we are bodies possessing a soul. I like to remember the philosophy of Saint Francis of Assisi. It is said that he called his body "Brother Donkey", and reminded his disciples to take care of their bodies, just as they would a beloved animal. This "donkey" we each are entrusted with, is a "gift" which carries our soul around, like a fine living vehicle. The body-vehicle is powered by nutrients from our air, food and water. Yet, undeniably, there is special rarified energy, which we can only envision and not truly describe. This energy, this spark of life, which was ignited in the body at the time of our conception, but existed long before the vehicle was manufactured in the womb of our mother, is classically called the "Eternal Soul". The light and energy of the soul is most evident in the chakras.

Historically the chakras have been described by most all traditions and cultures. Vedic tradition is an ancient religion,

c. 2000–1200 BC, of the Aryan peoples who entered northwestern India from Persia. It was the precursor of Hinduism, and its beliefs and practices are contained in the Vedas. The chakras are described in their ancient sacred books *Brahma Upanishad* and the *Yogatattva Upanashad*. The Sanskrit word *prana*, describes spiritual energy as breath. Breath, something all living beings possess, implies that spiritual energy is our birthright. Embryos and fetuses get their "breath", mainly oxygen, via the functions of the placenta.

The science of balancing the chakras gave rise to Ayurvedic medicine: a traditional Hindu system of healing based on the idea of balance in bodily systems, and uses diet, herbal treatment, yogic postures and breathing to maintain health.

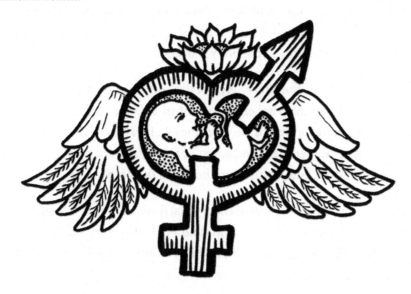

Tibetan Buddhism adapted the theory of chakras in the Vajrayana and Tantric traditions. Tantra describes the universal energy of creation known as "Kundalini" and defines the location of its concentrated potential as coiled at the base of our spines. The practice of Kundalini Yoga arouses this store of creative energy and causes it to rise up the pathway of the spinal column, stimulating each chakra along the way until union with the Divine is felt in the Sahasrara chakra, at the crown of the head.

Australian Aboriginal rock art, up to 6000 years old, depicts a rainbow serpent as the source of all life energy. This relates to the Kundalini tradition of knowledge, which states that energy is stored in a coiled snake at the base of our spines and rises up the chakras. (Note the relationship between the rainbow serpent and the umbilical cord.)

According to Frank Waters, author of *The Book of Hopi* (which describes native American folklore, ritual and migratory history), the Native American Hopi people believed that the human body was made with centers of vibration at the top of the head, in the brain, the throat, the heart, the naval, the genitals and the base of the spine.

In the Jewish mystical tradition, Kabbalah teaches that humans have concentrations of spiritual energy spheres. Spiritual achievement is attained when the spiritual energy in the body is balanced.

In Chinese medicine, the vital energy of the body is called Qi (it is also called Qi in Japan). When this vital energy is out-of-balance, depleted or stagnant, disease forms in the body and one becomes ill. Doctors of Chinese medicine have identified 12 meridians and some 365 acupuncture points, which they stimulate to restore flow, balance and health in the body.

Polynesians describe the spiritual energy that feeds our souls as Mana. Healers from Hawaii, Tahiti, Rapa Nui, Samoa and Fiji had special Mana, which they used along with massage, herbal remedies and bathing in both sweet stream and salty ocean water to help patients regain balance and restore their own Mana.

In Islam, universal life energy is called *Qudra* in Arabic. We also find similar awareness of seven points of maximum energy in the body, called *lata'if*. In his essay, *Islam and Spiritual Healing*, Sheik Hisham Alkabbani says, "The *lata'if* are the points of maximum energy intake and are very important focal points of balance within the energy system. Disease and illness occur if a *lata'if* is unbalanced."

In the practice of Sufism (the mystical system of Muslim ascetics), Zikr, a rhythmic movement or dance of balance, activates the energy centers in the body, facilitating the process of purification of the heart. The goal of Zikr is to harmonize the body as an instrument tuned to God's remembrance. Union of the two worlds is embedded within us and awakened through meditation, Zikr and prayer, whereby the pathway between the heart and brain becomes illuminated.

While working as a midwife and studying the chakras, I came to wonder why we as a species have come to the brink of self-destruction. In an epiphany of revelation one sleepless night of many births, I realized that there has been a grave misunderstanding of the very essentials concerning life on earth and how we, as Mother Earth's stewards, actually evolve. The missing link is the placenta. This precious chakra has been treated in modern times as nothing more than medical waste. With this degradation of the placenta, we witness the breakdown of the fiber of consciousness, of each individual's ability to evolve and of society's ability to function peacefully.

There is little, if any, hard-core scientific proof that hormones are the bridge between spirit and matter. I cannot prove that the placenta, the organ richest in hormones, is the forgotten chakra. Yet as a midwife I have watched what happens to human beings at birth, and I have listened and made connections that feel like answers. From the point of view of a midwife, mother, grandmother and crone, the miss-use of technology, separation of mother and baby and unkindness at birth causes this profound hurt and trauma. This trauma haunts our earthly existence, often taking a lifetime to heal, if ever. Jeannine Parvati, author of *Prenatal Yoga & Natural Childbirth*, *Hygieia: a Woman's Herbal* and *Conscious Conception: Elemental Journey through the Labyrinth of Sexuality* (with Rico Baker), said "Healing birth heals Mother Earth." It is my belief that original sin is birth trauma, because it determines how we as a species impact our environment. Thus, protecting children at birth will initiate a better world, with the potential for healing change, within one generation.

Our Chakra Map

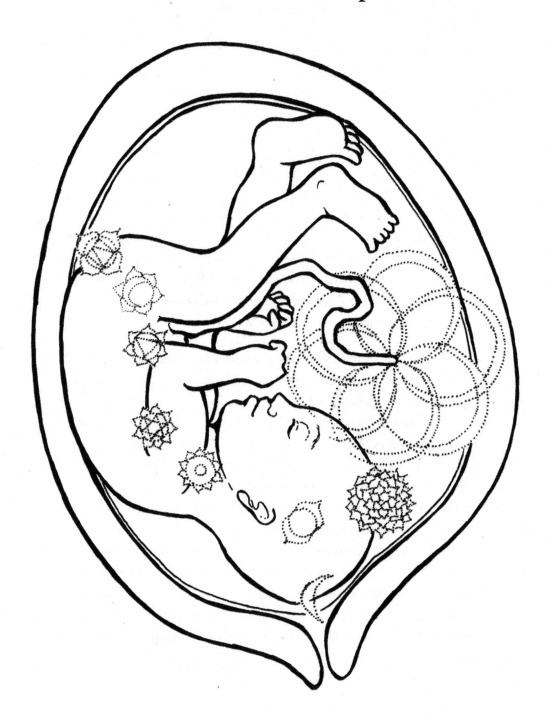

Sahasrara: Sun chakra - steers Kundalini energy - Unity Consciousness - BLISS - pineal gland - unites spirit with matter by oscillating in sync with Placenta Chakra – often perceived as a halo, CRYSTAL unity/separation.

 Bindu: Moon chakra - God Consciousness - NECTAR - hypothalamus - transcendent experience - VIOLET enthusiasm/apathy

 Ajna: 3rd Eye chakra - Intuition - PERCEPTION - pituitary gland - mid brain atop spinal column - muscles, body's control center - INDIGO comfort/pain.

 Vishuddhi: Throat chakra- Abundance - EXPRESSION - thyroid - articulation/self-actualization – OCEAN BLUE contentment/anger/forgiveness

 Anahata: Heart/love chakra - ACCEPTANCE - thymus - self esteem, the center of our Chakra system -GREEN courage/fear.

 Manipura: Will chakra- power - PARTICIPATION - naval radiating to spine nurturing our etheric body via the Solar Plexus, "Gut Feelings" pancreas/adreanals - YELLOW belonging/grief.

 Mooladhara: Root - survival - TRUST - male: perineum, female: cervix - physiological needs, excretion and sexuality - RED arousal/numbness.

 Swadhisthana: Sensation - the unconscious - VITALITY - base of spinal cord, sacral plexus of nerves and spleen - ORANGE safety/apathy.

 Apara: Placenta -origin -EPIPHANY - hormone bed/cord - bridge spirit/ matter conduit -RED, INDIGO, VIOLET, CRYSTAL unity/separation, mother/child matrix.

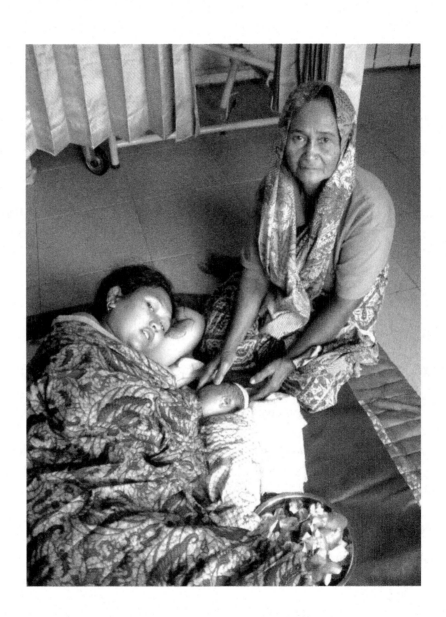

Placenta:
Our Hero/Heroine in Myth and History

From Ancient Sumeria to the Americas, Asia, Oceania, Aboriginal Australia, Medieval Europe and Africa, the placenta in myth and legend is both protector and monster to the enemies of her children. She is depicted as a dragon, angel, gazelle, deer, alligator, fish, tapir, frog, monkey, horned ox, turtle, lizard, wog, elephant, dog, lion, horned adder and cobra. She can be the Tree of Life, the stump representing the severed umbilical cord, or an eagle, raven, turkey, dove, vulture, hawk, man-bird, thunderbird or Phoenix. Sometimes in ancient stories the phallic symbols of snake, vine or rainbow are in actuality depicting the umbilical cord of the Placental Dragon, representing the creative power of reproduction.

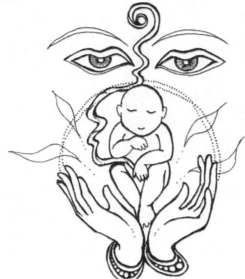

The placenta is also represented by images of angels. Solomon's temple was lined with cedar wood (considered the Tree of Life) from the garden of Ishtar, who was the Earth Mother in Lebanon. This sanctuary had only one entrance and exit – like a womb – and was said to be carved with images of the Tree of Life and the two-headed cherubim symbolizing the Placenta Monster Angel.

The Gorgon

Perhaps the image that most closely resembles our real placentas is the Gorgon: the three sisters in Greek Mythology, including Medusa, who had the power to turn people into stone. The Gorgon takes the form of a bodiless head with serpents for hair, like the placenta and umbilical cord, and has been depicted with claws, tusks, snakeskin and even angelic wings. Euripides (Athens 480-406 BC) wrote that Gaia, the earth goddess, created the Gorgon to protect her sons, mimicking the child-protecting function of the placenta.

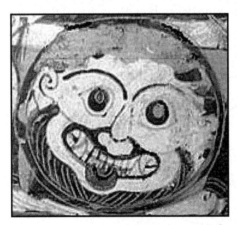

Protective Gorgon on the shield of Achilles at his burial by Thetis; Corinthian black-figure hydria, 560–550 BC - Louvre [1]

"Om Nana ketuet tanippoe!" A prayer chanted by Cunas Indians when afraid of the dark, imploring the Placenta Monster, "Holy Om Nana, do not make me sick tonight!"

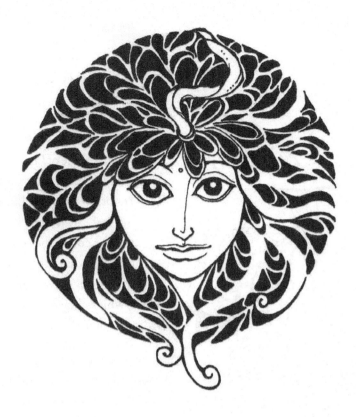

The Egyptian god of pleasure, Bes, dispelled evil spirits and was depicted as an obese dwarf, his lion-like face is reminiscent of the placenta. He protected children and women in labor and even assisted his wife, Taurt, with childbirth.

> *Come down, placenta, come down! I am Horus who conjures in order that she who is giving birth becomes better than she was, as if she was already delivered... Look, Hathor will lay her hand on her with an amulet of health! I am Horus who saves her!* – Excerpt from the birthing spell that was recited four times over the image of Bes[2]

Taurt was an Egyptian goddess and protector of fertility and childbirth and associated with the nursing of infants.[3] Her form: body of hippopotamus, tail of crocodile and feet of lion.[4] In Sumeria, a clay Khumbaba was used in childbirth as a protective totem. This wrinkled mask of Khumbaba is described in Assyrian-Babylonian legend as a replica of our placentas.

Totems

Totem poles, typically made from cedar trees, are most often associated with the Tree of Life. Totem poles stem from a native matriarchal tradition and were hollowed out so that salt water (like amniotic fluid) could be poured into them. Indian clans chose animals for their totems like bears, monkeys and birds, which they believed were born from the branches of the Tree of Life.

There was reverence for the individual's placenta but, like a placental family line, they also revered the placentas of past generations and considered them like Angels, protectors of the people.

Other animals depicted in placental totems include the tapir and deer for the Cunas Indians. In Southeast Asia, the white elephant holding a lotus flower with her trunk symbolizes the protector placenta and in Iran it is the horned viper.

In India the stag and the gazelle are honored as placental symbols, while the Pueblo Indians held the gopher turtle in high esteem for the same reason.

The Placental Dragon

The fourth Brahmana of Vedic text speaks of the Gonharva Visvavasu: the Rainbow Genius, Earth Mother's Placental Dragon.[5]

The Cuna Indians of Panama consider the coming-out party of a new woman the most essential ceremony for protecting her ability to mother children. They begin this ceremony by symbolically feeding the Earth Mother's Placental Dragon.[6] According to archaeologist, Sir John Marshall, the Naga people of northwest India were serpent worshipers. Their great ancestor was the god of wisdom. A teacher deity whose wisdom stemmed from his presence at the birth of the ocean: the release of the amniotic fluids of the Earth Mother.

For the Native American Indian tribes, this same dragon, released from the Earth Mother's womb and riding into birth on the ocean waters, is the protector of humankind. Later in history it became the Salmon of Wisdom for the Druids.[7]

The Incas and Sumerian kings as well as Mochica and Maya warriors wore the rainbow as a symbol. In their mythologies, the rainbow represents the Earth Mother's placenta and umbilical chord.[8] So, most likely, the rainbow was worn as a talisman to remind them of the Earth Mother's Placental Dragon, the totemic spirit that guards her children. According to the Potawatomis Indian legend the mole stole the Earth Mother's placental rainbow, but not before it gave rise to the colorful butterfly wings and bird feathers that we still enjoy today.

In a Native North American Pueblo story the Placental Dragon's head is cut off, which causes the "great flood" of salt water (amniotic fluid). The horns of the dragon's head are the Tree of Life. From this tree, also representing the placenta, grows the sacred vine depicting the umbilical cord.

The Tree of Life

The roots of trees draw moisture and nutrients from the Earth Mother, and then by way of precipitation, they deliver this life-giving water back to the earth's atmosphere – thus, the miracle of rain. At the same time, trees transpose carbon dioxide into life-sustaining oxygen. By rain and by air the trees also purify our environment. We see this relationship mirrored in the placentas of all higher mammals. Placentas are a joint venture between mother and child. It is these exact functions of delivering nutrients, moisture and oxygen, that sustain life on Earth, as well as life in the womb.

In India, visitors to sacred Bodhi trees hang a cord or cloth from it to symbolize the umbilical connection. The Maori Tuhoes people hang the naval cords of their babies in a locally designated Tree of Life. The Igarot mountain peoples of the Philippine Islands hang the placenta and cord of their babies high in trees. Beside the Ishtar gate of Babylon is a figure of the Placental Dragon, *Musshu*, his horns are the stump of the Tree of Life.[9] Perhaps the Menorah, branched candlestick, central to Jewish rituals, represents the tree of life. The prophet Jeremiah believed his vision of the almond tree, also a symbol of the Tree of Life, meant that God's word would quickly be fulfilled.

> The visionary Yoko Ono, inspired by temple wish trees from her childhood in Japan, installs modern day Trees of Life all over the world. People are encouraged to write their wishes on bits of paper and tie them to the Wish Trees. Yoko promises to collect these wishes from all over the world, she already has over 100,000, to include them in the "Imagine Peace Tower" she is making in Iceland.

I believe that the placenta is each person's Tree of Life. In Indonesia, *Kayon* means Tree of Life. The name *Kayon* comes from the word *kayu*, meaning wood. The *Kayon* is an archetypical symbol in Indonesia, essential in the shadow puppet theatre performance called *Wayang Kulit*, a traditional, ceremonial art form still strong throughout Southeast Asia.

In the *Wayang Kulit*, the puppets represent form while the shadows represent the soul. The soul is believed to be the most important part of existence so the shadow is the focus of the plays. I liken this to the placenta, as it too has both a living form and a soul. Soon after our birth, the body of the placenta dies, while its soul lives beside us in spirit as our shadow guardian.

The shadow representation of the *Kayon* (Tree of Life puppet) plays a significant role in Indonesian moral and spiritual instruction. It is meant to symbolize the life force ascending from mother to child and mirrored in the energetic exchange between the earth and the heavens through human beings, who serve as the bridge between them. In traditional *Wayang Kulit*, the three to six hour performance of mythical tales always opens with the *Kayon* puppet as the Tree of Life. It represents our roots, similar to our beginnings inside the womb with our placenta.

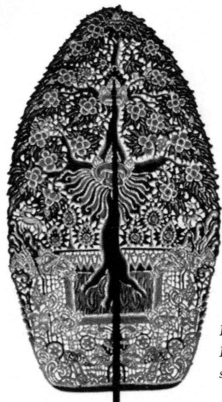

Kayon: a traditional Indonesian shadow puppet symbolizing the Tree of Life.

Ezekiel

In the Jewish, Islam and Christian religions, Ezekiel (Hebrew: יְחֶזְקֵאל, Yehezkel, Arabic: ذو الكفل) is revered as a prophet and priest who prophesied for about 22 years while exiled in Babylon sometime in the 6th century BC. Practicing Christians, Muslims and Jews who choose umbilical non-severance see passage 16:4 of the Book of Ezekiel as relevant to the strength and clarity of the visionary prophet:

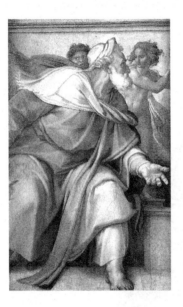

"As for your birth, on the day of your birth your cord was not cut and you were not washed in water to make you clean; you were not salted or folded in linen bands."
(16:4 Hebrews)

Historically, Ezekiel was condemned and, as the biblical text continues, the allegory becomes less understandable; yet, I must wonder at the significance of this passage. Though his condemners saw his uncut cord as punishment, I wonder if this non-severence led to his gift of psychic clarity, for Ezekiel became a revered prophet and visionary. Perhaps his punishment became the source of his ability and made him the remarkable religious figure that he is considered today.

Global Placenta Tales and Traditions

The Wand of Hippocrates, the Caduceus, symbol of medical science, also known as the heraldic staff belonging to Hermes, the Greek guardian of health, and also as the Wand of Mercury, messenger of the ancient Roman Gods, is what we recognize internationally as the universal symbol of doctors and healers. It is composed of two snakes wound around a central wand. This symbol is derived from the umbilical cord, which has three vessels: two arteries wound around a central vein. Both the symbol and the umbilical cord it was modeled after can be considered angels of healing, expressions of unity, peace and fertility.[10]

Native American Navajo tradition encourages the baby's grandmothers to bury their newborn grandchild's placenta and umbilical cord at a special place in the earth that represents their dreams for the child. Among the Hopi and many other Native American peoples it was traditionally believed that the first humans were born from the womb of the Earth Mother, attached to her placenta by the umbilical cord. The Earth Mother's placenta was said to be like a tribe or community that nourishes its individual children. Even the early pioneers of America were said to have practiced umbilical non-severance to prevent infection from the open wound of a cut cord.[11] In old Hawaii, the father of a new baby would bring the placenta to the ocean and leave it cradled in a *puka* (hole) in the volcanic stone by the sea. There the sacred organ could go home to her mother ocean.

In ancient Egyptian royal processions, the Pharaoh was preceded by his dried placenta held aloft on a pole, a symbol of his magical and spiritual power and leadership, which predated his birth. Commoners of Egypt would bury their children's placentas or throw them in the Nile. It has even been speculated that women of old Egypt ate a small bit of their placentas.[12]

Expectant Inuit Mothers avoid wearing rings or braids in their hair, because they believe it will cause the umbilical cord to be wrapped around the baby's neck. In Bolivia, mothers avoid knitting while pregnant to prevent the umbilical cord getting wrapped around the baby's neck. The Cunas, who originally lived in borderlands between Columbia and Peru, believed in a placenta spirit resembling a guardian dog that helped the child navigate his soul boat on the amniotic waters through the labyrinth toward earthly life. To protect new mothers from infection and postpartum cramping, a Costa Rican midwife may wrap the placenta in paper and bury it in a dry hole with ashes from the cooking fire.

In Guatemala, if the placenta is not born easily, a common remedy is to boil a purple onion in beer and have the woman drink the liquid. The midwives believe the placenta needs the heat of the newborn to deliver; If the cord is cut before the placenta is born, they believe that the placenta will rise into the throat of the mother and choke her. If she must cut the cord prior to the placenta delivering, the midwife ties it to the mother's leg with a strong stout string, using many knots to keep it from rising.

Mayan people's religious tradition roots them to the earth at the moment of birth. When a Mayan child is born, the placenta is buried in the ground as a religious ritual. This place holds special meaning for the Maya; it is where the individual is symbolically "planted" in the ground to root his or her Mayan identity. In this way the person will not become individualistic or selfish, but a part of the community, of nature and of the cosmos.[13]

In parts of Vietnam the placenta is traditionally buried under the mother's bed. Traditionally, in the Philippines, Indonesia, Laos and many other Asian cultures, a child born in the caul, the double-layered (amnion and chorion) placental sac, is said to have many gifts to share in life and that she may become a healer, or may have even been a monarch in a previous life. In Cambodia a spiky plant is placed over the carefully chosen placental burial site to ward off evil spirits and dogs from what the people believe is "the globe of the origin of the soul." In Nepal the placenta is said to be the baby's friend called the *bucha-co-satthi*. Childless women in Japan have been known to borrow the petticoat of a pregnant friend or relative and step over the burial site of a new placenta to gain fertility. The Hmong peoples of Southeast Asia consider the child's placenta her first and most significant 'jacket'. It is buried outdoors.

After death, each Hmong journeys back, retracing all her life's locations until she reaches the burial spot of her placenta.

Jane Goodall reported in her book, *In the Shadow of Man,* that in her long observation of chimpanzees in the wild, she found that they did not sever the umbilical cords of their babies.

The Maori of New Zealand traditionally respected the mother and child by keeping the placenta and the umbilical cord attached to the newborn baby. Colonizers discouraged this, and hospitals began burning the placenta. By the 1980s, the indigenous peoples of New Zealand were able to restore this important part of their culture so that the hospitals now return the placenta and umbilical cord to the mother if she so requests. The Maori call the placenta *whenua* and the umbilical cord *pito.* They believe that when the child's *whenua* and *pito* are buried on *Marae,* tribal land, the individual's sacred link with the Earth Mother *Papatuanuku* is cemented.[14]

Traditional Ukrainian midwives would look carefully at the newborn placenta to divine just how many children this mother was destined to have. The placenta could not be buried in a doorway, or the mother would become infertile.[15] Turkish parents will also bury the placenta, but if they wish for their child to be a devout Muslim, they bury the cord in the courtyard of a mosque. If they dream the child will be well educated, they may throw the baby's cord over a schoolyard wall.[16] To render himself infertile, a man in Transylvania, who had had quite enough children, would burn his newest baby's placenta and then mix it with ashes and water to drink.[17] Daughters of the Kwakiutl culture of British Columbia are said to become skilled clam diggers if their placentas are buried at the high-tide mark of the sea. Boys' placentas were left exposed to be eaten by ravens so that they would have prophetic vision.[18] Smiling Malaysian babies are said to be playing with their placentas.

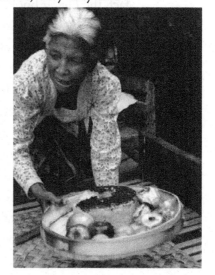

The Placenta in Bali

Where I make my home, in Bali, Indonesia, it is believed that the placenta, called *Ari-ari*, is the physical body of the child's guardian angel. While the physical body of the angel dies shortly after the baby is born, the angel's spirit stays with the child for his or her entire life. Each night the child bids goodnight to her *Ari-ari* and upon rising, she greets her placenta and thanks her for the protection the *Ari-ari* will provide for the coming day. At death, the human soul is accompanied into the afterlife by her placenta, steward of the mystery. There, the placenta goes with the soul and stands before the Gods and Goddesses to testify on behalf of her human twin. The *Ari-ari* tells the story of this person's life and, like a lawyer or advocate, defends this soul's actions, testifying as to whether she followed her Dharma (duty - promises made by the soul before birth) in life.

According to the *Lontar*, the sacred books of Bali Hindu Dharma, written in Sanskrit, the placenta must be strictly guarded. It was forbidden to cut the child's umbilical cord before the placenta was safely delivered, as they believed it would cause premature death of the placenta and a cascade of calamities. Ancient authors of the Bali *Lontar* books knew that the placenta still lives even after the baby is born, as evidenced by the pulsing arteries and vein. In fact, the *Lontar* books recommend that many hours be allowed to pass after the placenta's birth before placenta and baby are separated - if at all. In old Bali, it was unheard of to disrespect the natural life cycle of the placenta. If the cord was to be severed, a new sharpened blade made of bamboo was used, as metal knives were believed to harbor infections. A terrible punishment, in old Bali, even for adults, was to force one to go far away from the burial site of his placenta. This would cause extreme grief, and, if one stayed away too long, mental illness might set in. A family that moves house will take dirt from the graves of their children's placentas and ritually make a new placenta grave at the doorway of the new house. Sadly, in modern Bali, where births most often occur in hospitals, the cord is clamped and cut immediately: a Western medical protocol exported to the East, with grave cultural impact.[19]

Balinese women today still make offerings for the placenta. Soon after the cord of the baby is either cut or burned, the father and his closest male relatives honor and bury the *Ari-ari*. It is entombed in a coconut, wrapped in sacred white cloth, which is then wrapped in the black fiber of sago palm. A boy's placenta will be buried on the right side of the door of the family home and the girl's on the left. Buried with the *Ari-ari* are bits of paper inscribed with Sanskrit prayers and wishes, as well as a pinch of life sustaining rice, fragrant flowers and holy water. Finally, a stone is placed on top of the grave.

If a Balinese mother's milk is scant, she may collect some dirt from the *Ari-ari's* burial site and rub it on her breasts. Before taking a long journey with the baby, the mother will place a small offering on a stone over the placenta's grave and drip a few drops of her milk there. Some families place a paintbrush in the burial hole of the placenta to insure the child will be artistic. If the family

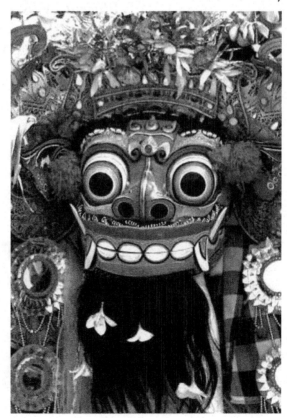

desires that this child be adept at writing, they may throw a pen into the hole. My son's placenta was buried with a guitar pick, and, indeed, he is very musical! For the first seven days, a candle, lantern or electric bulb burns all night at the gravesite of the placenta. For the next several years, every full moon, new moon and *Kajeng Kliwon* (Balinese day of demon cleansing), the child's placenta is given offerings.

Creation Myth

The Mandinka people of southern Mali believe that a piece of the placenta from the "Great Mother's" womb was thrown down and became the earth, the rest of the placenta became the sun.[20] An ancient Babylonian creation story casts the Milky Way as amniotic fluid – 3,000 B.C.[21] In West Africa, the Fans believe that God created the first human out of clay in the form of a lizard, which I believe is meant to represent male sperm. The creator put this first lizard into a pool, the womb of the Earth Mother. At the end of seven sacred days the being was called forth and born human, the lizard became the Placental Dragon.[22]

Placenta Vessels

In Germany, pottery vessels dating from the 16th to the 19th centuries A.D were found by a scientist from the University of Tubingen. The pots were buried in groups, sometimes up to 50 together, and traces of human placenta were found inside. Local folklore of that time in Germany suggested that to bury a baby's placenta in such a pot would ensure the health and well-being of the child.[23] In Indonesia, the placenta is commonly buried or put to sea in a coconut or a clay pot. Hospitals would not dream of throwing away the placenta: It is always given to the family for disposal according to their cultural traditions.

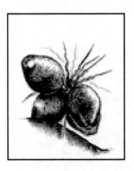

Coconut, the most common placenta vessel in SE Asia.

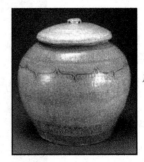

Korean placenta jar from antiquity

Buddhist Lore

Gautama Buddha and the great Tibetan Buddhist Avatar,
Padmasambhava known as Guru Rinpoche were called "Lotus Born".

The placenta god, *Ena Kōjin*, has the job of protecting and nurturing babies. It becomes *Gushō Jin*, the guardian spirit and silent witness to our day-to-day thoughts and acts. In a sense, it is our identical twin, a doppelganger following our birth, invisible to us, but closer and more honest to our essential selves. The *Ena Kōjin* appears as a peaceful Buddha to those who are virtuous and as a wrathful demon to people living outside of integrity.[24]

Daruma, also known as Bodhidharma, is said to be the father of Zen Buddhism. He is known for his red robes, red being the color that wards off disease. The Daruma Doll, a symbol of good luck and healing, is believed to be a placenta deity. It is called upon to make couples fertile and to ease childbirth. Zen Buddhist parents dress their sick children in red and will often give them a Daruma doll, calling upon the spirit of the placenta to speed recovery. There is also a Japanese story that tells of an imperial prince, Shotoku Taishi (547 – 622 AD) born in a stable, like Jesus. On the occasion of his special birth,

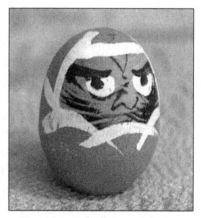

Daruma ~ Bodhidharma ~ Placenta

it is said that the Boddhidharma wished to be present, so he reincarnated as a horse and neighed three times. His presence at birth reinforces the belief that Bodhidharma, or Daruma, is the placenta deity.

In Tibet, the placenta is saved until an astrologer indicates the first auspicious day for the father or other close relatives to bury it. It may be buried anywhere as long as no animals can dig it up. The placenta is wrapped in clean cloth and buried deep in the ground, often the children of the family assist. The burial place is not marked, but the process of burying it symbolizes respect for the placenta, which nourished the baby in the womb. The umbilical cord is kept in a safe place in the house for about a year. The mother uses the cord to heal thrush in the baby's mouth by dipping it in milk, tea, or water and rubbing it over the sore.[25]

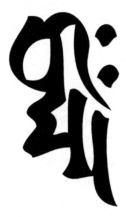

Immediately after a child's birth, as soon as its mouth is opened, the symbol *Dhih* is painted in saffron powder on the newborn's tongue. *Dhih* is the seed syllable of *Manjusri*, the deity of wisdom. They do this so the baby will grow to be wise and well spoken, highly valued in the rooftop of the world. In some parts of Tibet, the *Dhih* is believed to give the child intelligence, longevity, and good fortune. Some Tibetan families put blessed butter, which has been prayed over, on the baby's tongue. It symbolizes good health, longevity, and always having enough to eat.

The Placenta in Turkey

The Placenta in Turkey is called: "Es". Es means partner, like a husband or a wife. It comes from the word: "Esit" which means "equal." Thus the placenta is your Equal Partner.

Traditionally the parents of a new baby would bury the child's placenta in their home garden. More recently the hospitals dispose of the placentas. so in the cities of Turkey today the parents will bury the baby's umbilical cord stump (after it falls away) in a significant place. For example, if the family wishes for the child to be a scholar, the cord stump would be buried at a university. Parents who wish their son to become a soldier will placed the umbilical stump on a military base. Farming families will bury the cord stump on the farm, etc. *Many thanks to Dr. Gulinihal (Rose Bush) & Dr. Hulya (Day Dream).*

Apara – Placenta of Vishnu the Protector

Lord Vishnu and his consort, the Goddess Lakshmi, along with Garuda, the eagle he rides, reclined on the coiled body of Ananta-sesha, the serpent of time. Together they rested in the tranquil amniotic primeval waters where, inside of them, lay all that once was, is, and ever will exist: before form and identity. This was called Yoga-nidra, the cosmic slumber, or pregnancy. At birth Vishnu opened his eyes and then, connected by the umbilical cord from his naval, his placenta was born - his twin, Brahma the Creator and Shiva, his *lingam* (penis), sitting upon a lotus with a thousand petals.

Following his birth, Vishnu's preserving, restoring, and protecting powers manifested in the world as the ten earthly incarnations known as avatars. The avatars arrive either to prevent a great evil or to effect good upon the earth. The ten avatars of Lord Vishnu are Matsya the fish (mermaid or merman), Kurma the turtle (who the Balinese Hindus believe their world sits upon), Varaha the boar, Narasimha (half man half lion), Vamana the dwarf, Parashurama the Brahmin, Rama the hero (who teaches us of love between husband and wife), Krishna the cow herder, Buddha the enlightened one and Kalki the horse (yet to come to the earth). Hindu prophets say that it is the coming of Kalki that may save our ailing environment from utter destruction.

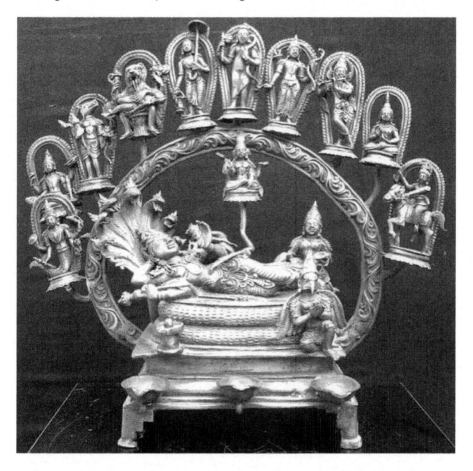

This bronze sculpture from Bangladesh depicts the story of the birth of Brahma from the navel of Vishnu. Brahma is the placenta of Vishnu from which all the incarnations of Vishnu then arise.

When I am asked,
"Why don't you cut babies' umbilical cords?"

I say, "Isn't the real question: Why do you cut?"

It's interesting that those of us on the path of nonviolence
are being asked to justify our peaceful non-interventions,
by the perpetrators of intemperate protocols.

~ Ibu Robin Lim, CPM

Modern vs Traditional Treatment of the Placenta

If you were born in a hospital in North America, Europe or the so-called "developed" or "civilized" world, your placenta was labeled medical waste and incinerated. It was treated as garbage and thrown away without ritual or even a pause to offer gratitude for its significant role in your advent. In the past, some hospitals would sell their patients' placentas to cosmetic companies. Without your permission, your placenta may have ended up in a shampoo or facial cream product.

In 1994 it was discovered that approximately 360 tons of human placenta was being sold by hospitals annually to French pharmaceutical companies, who used it to make the protein Albumin. None of the families of the babies to whom the placenta's belonged were aware of the commercial use of their placentas. None of them had agreed to share their genetic flesh and blood commercially. That same year Britain banned the practice of collecting and marketing the placentas of unsuspecting citizens.[1]

For many indigenous peoples of the world, this is shocking and tragic. In Indonesia, when people ask me what happened to my placenta, and I tell them that it was most likely disposed of by the military hospital where I was born, they weep for me. A hospital in Indonesia that does not respectfully give the placenta to the baby's family risks outrage from the parents and their community. Indonesian families quickly bring the placenta home and perform important rituals, essential to the baby's future well being.

I recall attending the birth of a young single mother, Megan, who required a cesarean birth for her baby, Corwin. She had intended to have a home birth but instead needed to be transported from her home to the hospital. Megan was broken-hearted that her baby boy's placenta would be treated as medical waste and thrown away. At the hospital I spoke with Megan's attending nurse, who was kind, loving and sympathetic to Megan's concern for her placenta. She told me of the hospital protocol and together we wondered if their policy to restrict families from taking home their placentas was based in law or prejudice.

Later that evening, as I was leaving the hospital with Megan's mother, we were delighted to find Corwin's placenta wrapped in a double plastic bag, waiting for us in the front seat of the car. The note attached said only, "Shhhh."

> *"Another thing very injurious to the child, is the tying and cutting of the navel string too soon; which should always be left till the child has not only repeatedly breathed but till all pulsation in the cord ceases. As otherwise the child is much weaker than it ought to be, a portion of the blood being left in the placenta, which ought to have been in the child."*
> – Erasmus Darwin, (Charles Darwin's grandfather) *Zoonomia*, 1801

More than two centuries ago doctors like Darwin began questioning the immediate cutting of the cord which had become fashionable protocol, even habit, among medical birth attendants. The practice of severing the mother-placenta-child connection quickly and clinically came into practice only after men took over the management of birth. Today midwives and doctors are still questioning the wisdom of early umbilical cord clamping and cutting. On August 1st, 2010, Dr. Kornia SpOG, specialist of Obstetrics and Gynecology at Udayana University in Denpasar, Bali, Indonesia, gave a seminar supporting the choice of Lotus Birth (umbilical cord non-severance) and delayed clamping and cutting of the umbilical cord. He assured the audience that it was safe and that choosing to leave the umbilical cord intact was a human right. A year earlier his colleague SpOG, Dr. Hariyasa Sanjaya left his own newborn daughter's umbilical cord intact after her cesarean birth. To my knowledge this baby, Gayatri, was the first child of an obstetrical surgeon to have a Lotus Birth.

Prior to the medical establisment's agresive takeover of birth, midwives, nurses, traditional birth attendants, grandmothers, good neighbors, any woman helping a woman birth would wait patiently before separating the reproductive trinity. In traditional cultures the neighborhood witch-midwife used her knowledge of herbs, massage and wisdom to mend the sick and injured, and in attending birthing mothers. She (in some cultures 'he' as was sometimes the case in Bali) would help the family clean up and wash linens after the birth. Someone would cook a meal, feed the mother and all in attendance would partake in celebrating the newly arrived baby. They would sit by the fire and discuss possible names for the baby. After hours of slow whispered talk and storytelling it would be time for the midwife to go home and only then would they think about severing the umbilical cord. Until then, the placenta with the cord intact was tucked in beside the mother while the baby nursed at her breast and the mother rested and bonded with her newborn.

Quite often, the traditional midwife might be called away to attend another birth, to minister to a dying soul, or help a neighbor find a missing goat, and the placenta-cord-baby trinity would be left intact another day, or just left until it naturally released. This was not a problem, for fear based medical protocols had not yet infiltrated the hearts and minds of the people. The placenta was just a natural part of the baby.

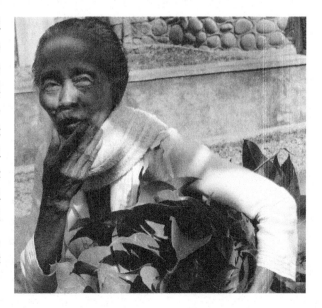

Cord Cutting

"We must keep in mind that cord cutting is originally a ritual inseparable from myth (eg, the widespread belief that the colostrum is harmful) that leads to early mother–newborn separation. If it were possible to neutralize the effects of such deep-rooted beliefs and rituals, there would be no excuse to separate the neonate from the mother." – Michel Odent

In this day and age we all understand the importance of a strong immune system. Viruses, including HIV/AIDS, and the increasing prevalence of life-threatening cancers are real, daily threats to our lives. Yet, our immune systems are denied a fighting chance from birth due to the widely accepted protocols of medical practice that call for immediate clamping and cutting of the umbilical cord and separation of mother and child immediately after birth. These two practices, in addition to the use of anesthesia in labor, which can be a cocktail of drugs (including narcotics) that cross the maternal-placental barrier into the baby, cause serious damage to our immune and endocrine systems from the very beginning of our lives.

In hospitals and in some birthing centers, all over the planet, these insensitive protocols also result in the babies being whisked immediately away from their mothers to be evaluated, weighed, measured, bathed and dressed before they are returned. This tragically compromises the natural maternal-infant bonding and breastfeeding, and also increases the likelihood of postpartum hemorrhage; as the initiation of breastfeeding within the first minutes of a baby's life helps contract the uterus and prevent excessive maternal bleeding.

"... Immediate cord clamping is clearly identified as a cause of newborn neurological (brain) injury ranging from neonatal death through cerebral palsy to mental retardation and behavioral disorders. Immediate cord clamping has become increasingly common in obstetrical practice over the past 20 years; today, rates of behavioral disorders (e.g., ADD/ADHD) and developmental disorders (e.g., autism, Asperger's, etc) continue to climb and are not uncommon in grade school."

– George M. Morley, M.B., Ch. B., FACOG [2]

Even when an oxytocic medication is required to control maternal hemorrhage, I leave the baby's umbilical cord intact for as long as three hours or more, and I have observed no ill side effects for mother or child. In addition, recent research conducted in this area supports late clamping, because it may prevent iron deficiency anemia in childhood, which is of special importance in developing countries (Michaelsen et al 1995, Pisacane 1996). I believe that, presently, there is sufficient evidence to justify saying that for nearly all babies, delayed umbilical cord clamping and cutting or no umbilical cord severance is beneficial.

> *"It is common practice nowadays for the cord to be doubly clamped while the child is on the mother's abdomen and the scissors are handed to the parents to complete the job. Most mothers refuse, leaving it to the husband; some mothers recoil in horror, and if the cord is left intact, most mothers will not touch it. If they do, and especially if it is pulsating, the cord is treated as gently and tenderly as is a tiny finger or an ear of the child. New mothers are strongly inhibited from damaging the cord."*
> – Dr. G. M. Morley [3]

For a long time, doctors, scientists, midwives, doulas, parents and many others have been questioning the practice of clamping and cutting of babies' umbilical cords, wondering: Is clamping and cutting the umbilical cord really necessary? Pioneer midwives like Jeannine Parvati, Mary Kroeger and Ina May Gaskin advise against these unnecessary medical protocols, as do I.

Prior to 1995, I cut cords hundreds of times. I waited until the cord seemed to stop pulsing, but that felt uncomfortable in my heart. I felt like I was shutting off my feelings for the baby and mother, to enable myself to cut the cord. Too often I heard the babies cry out, flinch or clench their fists at the moment of the cut. In 1985, while pregnant with my third child, Zhouie, I read about Jeannine Parvati Baker's lotus births. I was moved, but I couldn't imagine that I could accomplish this kind of patience. When I mentioned it to my own midwife (now deceased), she laughed and assured me that it would in fact be too inconvenient. I let the idea go at the time, and she cut my baby's cord. I would birth two more babies, but I was not ready to look that deeply into my own process. Today, it is the one thing I would change about the births of my own children. When my granddaughter was born, we waited many hours before severing her umbilical cord. When my grandson Bodhi was born, he was left intact until his umbilical cord released spontaneously, a full Lotus born baby.

When my first child Déjà was born, I chose to birth her at home and we cut her umbilical cord after only 2 hours. Twenty-four years later, Déjà, who was by then a grown woman, was in a panic: "I've lost my purse! Mother, help me, I'll die without my purse!" Déjà's purse was oval shaped, weighing about a pound, brown-red in color and had a long strap. It reminded me even then of a placenta. Misplacing it caused her to panic and cry. Moments after Déjà cried, "I'll die without my purse!" our eyes met in a moment of "a-ha." She laughed out loud and said, "This is all your fault mother. You never should have let my cord be cut." We hugged and one of Déjà's brothers unearthed the essential purse, the surrogate placenta. Déjà laughed when she realized she would not die without her purse, yet I can't shake the memory of her recoiling when her cord was cut as a newborn.

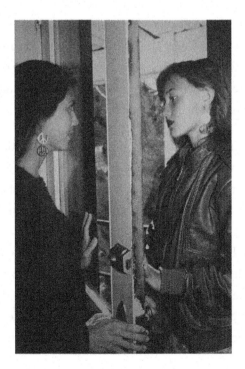

Neonatal Tetanus,
the Problem, the Solution...

"Tetanus is acquired when the spores of the bacterium Clostridium Tetani infect a wound or the umbilical stump. Spores are universally present in the soil. People of all ages can get tetanus but the disease is particularly common and serious in newborn babies ("neonatal tetanus"). It requires treatment in a medical facility, often in a referral hospital. Neonatal tetanus, which is mostly fatal, is particularly common in rural areas where deliveries are at home without adequate sterile procedures. WHO estimated that neonatal tetanus killed about 180 000 babies in 2002." [4]

Neonatal deaths from tetanus have been blamed on rural homebirths. Yet I have seen it happen following hospital deliveries, particularly in hospitals that are crowded and in an uproar, after natural disasters like earthquakes and tsunamis. However, tetanus can happen to any baby in any country, if the umbilical cord is cut. Early clamping and cutting of the umbilical cord puts any baby at risk.

Michel Odent in his succinct article for the *Lancet* makes the point perfectly: neonatal tetanus, a killer, is preventabl, if the umbilical cords of newborn babies are left intact for only a few hours. In S.E. Asia there has been an attempt to train traditional birth attendants in medical protocol; immediate clamping and cutting, and for this they were given a pair of scissors. This little bit of technology has caused an untold number of babies to die. Even medically trained midwives and doctors sometimes do not have adequately sterilized instruments. The best cure for tetanus is prevention, just leave the babies umbilical cords be. In the words of Dr. Odent...

"In their Seminar about maternal and neonatal tetanus (Dec 8, p 1947)[5], Martha Roper and colleagues present neonatal tetanus as a consequence of unsafe umbilical cord care practices. It should rather be presented as a complication of an intervention—ie, early cord cutting. If there is no rush to intervene, some hours later the cord is thin, dry, hard, and exsanguine. Then, it can be cut without any need for cord care practices. The risk of neonatal tetanus is eliminated.

We must keep in mind that cord cutting is originally a ritual inseparable from myths (eg, the widespread belief that the colostrum is harmful) that lead to early mother—newborn separation. If it were possible to neutralise the effects of such deep-rooted beliefs and rituals, there would be no excuse to separate the neonate from the mother. Apart from the prevention of neonatal tetanus, one might expect a cascade of secondary outcomes (higher haematocrit, immediate contamination of the neonate by germs satellite of the mother, early consumption of colostrum, effects on how the gut flora is established, etc).

At a time when global action is the watchword, one can wonder how cost effective it would be to teach the world that cutting the cord can wait many hours, that the neonate needs first its mother's arms and can find the breast during the hour after birth, and that the colostrum is precious. Our objective is not to discuss the particular case of wealthy countries where neonatal tetanus is almost unknown and drugless childbirth rare. I declare that I have no conflict of interest." [6]

Where I live in Indonesia, skilled, educated midwives are forced by the Departments of Health in their regions to clamp and cut the umbilical cords of babies two minutes after birth! [7] Why, given the clear risks of early cord clamping and cutting? Because JHPIEGO Corporation, an affiliate of John

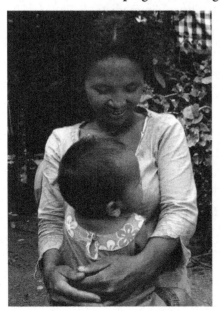

Hopkins University in Baltimore, USA, working along with the National Clinical Training Network [8] has implemented these recommendations as part of their maternal and child health integrated program. The publication and distribution of these protocols was made with the support of USAID, which, if you are an American, you are paying to perpetuate the early clamping and cutting of umbilical cords in many parts of the world. In my opinion, these corporations are educating well meaning midwives in protocols which were developed and implemented based on the medical myth that early clamping and cutting of the cord is indicated and safe.

"Delaying clamping the umbilical cord for a slightly longer period of time allows more umbilical cord blood volume to transfer from mother to infant and, with that critical period extended, many good physiological "gifts" are transferred through 'nature's first stem cell transplant' occurring at birth."
– Mankind's first natural stem cell transplant, Journal of Cellular and Molecular Medicine, 2010 [9]

Full Lotus Birth, which involves leaving the umbilical cord intact until it dries out and releases naturally (typically 3 to 9 days), is the ideal model of non-intervention and non-violence. It's a good option for those who wish to avoid unnecessary medical protocols.[10] I believe that waiting for the placenta to be born, so that the family sees the baby with the cord and placenta intact, is already a Lotus Birth and that 99% of the benefits are already had by the baby in the first minutes and hours following such a birth. However, I love the sight and feeling of an intact baby so much (a baby with its umbilical cord still connected), that I prefer full Lotus Birth. I have witnessed many families, who had not planned a full Lotus Birth, decide to leave the baby's umbilical cord intact, because once they see their beautiful child with his or her placenta, it feels strange to them to sever it. Some mothers of babies I have received, who had chosen a Lotus Birth, reported their children were like super-humans and that, as they grew, they spoke of the past and future as if they were there, transcending the linear concept of time. I am quick to point out that these children are not "super" but normal.

Some families may find full Lotus Birth burdensome. They are uncomfortable sleeping with a newborn baby still connected with its umbilical cord and placenta. For families who wish to wait a few hours, or can wait a day before gently severing the umbilical cord, there is a wonderful alternative to cord cutting: cord burning.

Cord burning was practiced in old China and was believed to help the Qi (Chi), latent in the placenta, move into the baby. Midwives have witnessed babies with dusky blue complexions and low APGAR scores* pink right up as the cord

---

* Test given to newborns immediately after birth to determine their physical condition: Activity, Pulse, Grimace, Appearance, and Respiration.

is burned. According to Bobbie Aqua, Doctor of Chinese Medicine, "Cord burning brings the element of fire to the birth. Warmth is essential for a baby's well-being and mother's recovery to full strength and ample milk supply."

When Yayasan Bumi Sehat (Healthy Mother Earth Foundation) was asked to join medical relief efforts in Aceh, Sumatra, Indonesia, the area hardest hit by the Dec. 26, 2004 earthquake and tsunami, we were forced to take a long look at the practice of cord cutting, due to a lack of sterile medical supplies. Midwives and traditional birth attendants (*dukun bayi* in Indonesian) in Aceh were faced with devastating loss. Many midwives lost their lives, as between 30% and 90% of the population in coastal villages perished within a couple of hours. The survivors were homeless. The fact that the surviving birth attendants had no instruments was secondary to the fact that they had no water to sterilize the instruments they had left. They had no cooking pots, no fuel for heating and no possible way to keep instruments sterile. It would have been foolish for us to provide them with scissors for umbilical cord cutting.

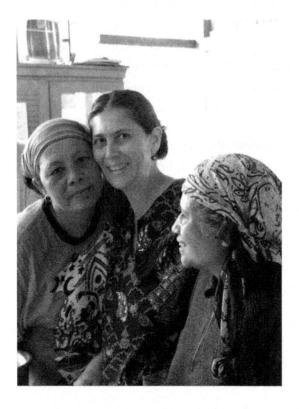

In our first week in Aceh, we met with 46 midwives and instructed them on how to burn umbilical cords, which eliminated their dependency on these now scarce resources. All of them were excited and relieved to learn a safer, more practical method of cord care. Everyone we met in Aceh had lost children, parents, husbands, or siblings. Yet the miracle of birth continued to unfold. A large percentage of the pregnant women died, as they could not outrun the tsunami, but with this method of cord severing now available to them, the survivors continued having their babies more safely.

While in Aceh after the tsunami, I encountered the miraculous birth story of Ibu Sarjani. She lost her first baby to tetanus infection caused by cutting her newborn daughter's umbilical with rusty scissors. Her second and third daughters perished in the tsunami, torn from her and her husband's arms. As Ibu Sarjani surrendered to death under the tsunami water, a caribou nudged her with her horn, which she instinctively grabbed. This sweet water buffalo swam to the surface, allowing Ibu Sarjani to climb onto the roof of the mosque, which was now at the level of the water. Miraculously, she also found her husband there.

That very night on top of the mosque (the only building in that village left standing), 70 other people also found refuge, everyone else in the village had perished. Ibu Sarjani went into labor. In what would turn out to be an unbelievable blessing, one of the other survivors on that roof was a midwife!

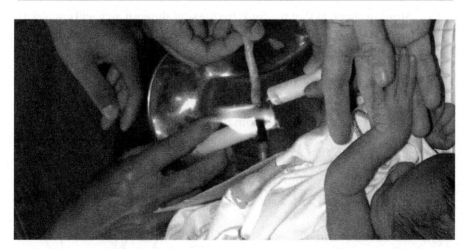

When the Bumi Sehat Disaster Relief Reproductive Health Team arrived in Haiti soon after the 2010 earthquake, they used cord burning as the safest way to sever umbilical cords following birth in hospitals that had been reduced to rubble and with no running water.[12]

Burning the Cord Instructions

If you do not have sterile instruments for cutting the umbilical cord, it is safer and cleaner to burn the cord. In addition, the cord stump will dry up and fall off faster if it is burned. Below are my instructions, which I advise you to follow carefully. Also, cord burning is best done with two people helping each other. It takes about ten to fifteen minutes. Cord burning may be done provided there are no regulations prohibiting this procedure in your area.

What you will need

- Two or more long candles
- A lighter or matches
- Heat guard, like cardboard – I use two layers
- A metal plate, kidney bowl or banana leaves to catch the wax

What you will not need

- Medicines (i.e. anti-infectives, alcohol, betadine, as fire cauterizes the cord stump making it sterile)
- String or clamp to shut the cord (the fire seals the cord, so it will not bleed)

Instructions

Unless this is an emergency procedure, it's best to wait three hours or more after the brith of the placenta. You may even wish to wait until the next morning to separate the placenta from the baby. There is no hurry.

The baby should be swaddled and lying on his or her side with the placenta lying opposite to the direction the baby is facing. Use a heat guard to protect the baby (i.e. cardboard with a slit in it).

Light two candles and choose a spot to burn the cord – about 10-12 cm (4 in.) from the baby's belly. Someone can hold the cord steady, but don't pull it too hard, be gentle.

Position the candles opposite one another, above the kidney bowl or plate to catch the melting wax, and begin burning the cord. As you begin to burn the cord you may hear a loud pop or explosion, which may even blow out your candles. Don't be alarmed. It is a natural sound, caused by the build up of gasses, and it means everything is working fine. Relight the candles and continue to burn the cord until it burns through.

While burning you may wish to turn the cord, roasting it all around. The smell is like barbecue. Keep burning until the cord has burned through totally. I suggest singing a spiritual song during this lovely fire ritual. From time to time, feel the cord on the baby's side of the heat guards, to make sure it is not getting too hot.

Once the cord and placenta are separated from the baby, wait some time before letting the burned cord stump touch the baby's skin. Check to the touch, as it may stay hot for a minute or two. You will not need to put any kind of medicine on the baby's cord stump. It will fall off in a few days all by itself. I have observed that the stumps of umbilical cords that have been burned seem to dry up and fall away more quickly than those that have been cut.

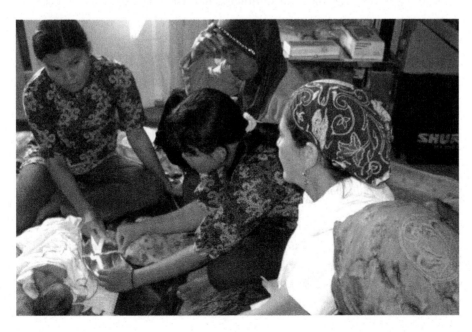

Cord Cutting and Disease

Some medical professionals believe that delayed umbilical cord clamping causes jaundice in babies. They assume and fear that keeping the umbilical cord attached will cause too much blood to flow into the baby, increasing the likelihood of jaundice. Thus, these medical professionals believe, erroneously, that they must control the amount of blood that flows into the baby after birth by immediately clamping and cutting the umbilical cord to prevent the risk of jaundice. In reality, the umbilical cord closes on its own when the baby receives the proper amount of blood. This being the case, there is no need for human intervention of the cord's natural blood transfer.

In order to understand this controversy better, you need to understand exactly what newborn jaundice is. One of the most important facts is that there are two kinds of jaundice: pathological and physiological. Physiological jaundice naturally occurs in many newborn babies. This non-life threatening type of jaundice is like an extension of the birth process, part of the physical changes that the baby goes through gradually as her body adjusts to life outside the womb. Typically physiological jaundice is described like this:

> *"Bilirubin is a yellow pigment that's created in the body during the normal recycling of old red blood cells. The liver processes bilirubin in the blood so that it can be removed from the body via the stool.*
>
> *Before birth, the placenta – the organ that nourishes the developing baby – removes the bilirubin from the infant so that it can be processed by the mother's liver. Immediately after birth, the baby's own liver begins to take over the job, but it can take time for the newborn liver to become fully functional. Therefore, bilirubin levels in an infant are normally a little higher after birth.*
>
> *High levels of bilirubin in the body can cause the skin to look yellow. This is called jaundice. Jaundice is present to some degree in most newborns. Such "physiological jaundice" usually appears between day 2 and 3, peaks between days 2 and 4, and clears by 2 weeks. Physiological jaundice usually causes no problems."* [11]

Pathological jaundice occurs under several conditions, including an incompatibility between the baby's and the mother's blood types, incompatibility of additional blood factors, or liver problems. The baby will display symptoms of listlessness, may run a fever, become disinterested in feeding and show a yellowing of its skin. It is important to have your baby checked if she shows any of these symptoms, as she will need phototherapy (using blue light to help clear excessive bilirubin from the baby's body) under the guidance of a pediatric specialist.

In the evolution of obstetric protocol (which was mostly designed and implemented by men), doctors became concerned with the prevention of jaundice. Their solution was immediate clamping and cutting of the umbilical cord to reduce the babies' blood volume, thus presumably reducing the incidence of jaundice. However, they neglected to weigh the consequences of this intervention, as denying newborns their full supply of cord blood can result in newborn anemia and a cascade of other conditions related to an inadequate supply of blood.

> *"Almost every baby lying in a hospital crib today and receiving phototherapy has been subject to this harsh protocol of immediate cord clamping and cutting. Doesn't it seem strange that it's efficacy has never been questioned."* – Wil Hemmerle, an outraged father

In an article published in *Pediatrics*, the official journal of the American Academy of Pediatrics, the authors found no increased threat of neonatal jaundice from late clamping and cutting of the cord: [12]

> *"Delayed cord clamping at birth increases neonatal mean venous hematocrit within a physiologic range. Neither significant differences nor harmful effects were observed among groups. Furthermore, this intervention seems to reduce the rate of neonatal anemia. This practice has been shown to be safe and should be implemented to increase neonatal iron storage at birth."*

Furthermore, Dr. Sarah Buckley also reveals in her well-researched article, *A Natural Approach to the Third Stage of Labour*, that there is no increased risk of jaundice in healthy babies when cord cutting is delayed:

> *"Some studies have shown an increased risk of polycythemia (more red blood cells in the blood) and jaundice when the cord is clamped later. Polycythemia may be beneficial, in that more red cells means more oxygen being delivered to the tissues. The risk that polycythemia will cause the blood to become too thick (hyperviscosity syndrome), which is often used as an argument against delayed cord clamping, seems to be negligible in healthy babies."*

Rh- Mothers, Babies and Placentas

In addition to the blood groups (A, B, O, AB), the Rh factor is written as either positive (present) or negative (absent). Most people are Rh positive (approx. 85%). This factor is normally of no concern, except during pregnancy. In some cases, either at the time of a miscarriage or the birth of an Rh+ baby, an Rh- mother may develop antibodies that cause her blood to combat the blood of subsequent Rh+ babies.

Women with Rh factor negative blood types may run a more frequent risk of developing antibodies against Rh positive blood at the time she gives birth if her baby's umbilical cord is immediately clamped and cut. When the umbilical cord of a newborn baby is immediately clamped, blood engorgement that takes place in the cord and placenta can put a strain on the complex vascular barrier between the mother and baby's circulatory systems. If a sufficient amount of time was not allowed to deliver all the blood to the baby, some of which is still in the cord and placenta, this strain can cause the baby's blood to mix with the mother's blood supply. This mixing causes her immune response to make antibodies against the foreign Rh+ blood. Rh sensitization endangers subsequent Rh+ children that an Rh- mom may bear.

In an article published in Mothering magazine in 1986 Author Hilary Butler states:

> *"For mothers who are Rh-negative, this [delayed cord severance] is especially important. Fewer Rh-negative mothers of Rh-positive babies develop antibodies when the cord is unclamped and separation of the placenta is spontaneous. Normally, the placental barrier prevents mixing of maternal and foetal circulation. However, when the placenta separates after cord clamping, the baby's blood, which is still in the placenta, can mix with the mother's blood, causing maternal contamination."*

> *"In Rh-negative women, many people believe that it is the clamping of a pulsing cord that causes the blood of the baby to transfuse into the blood stream of the mother causing sensitization problems. Robert S Mendelsohn, M.D., in his book 'How to Have a Healthy Child. . . In Spite of Your Doctor' blames the Rh neg problem on too quick clamping of the cord. Especially in Rh neg mothers I urge midwives to wait until the placenta is out before thinking about cord clamping."* – Gloria LeMay

Delaying the clamping and cutting of the umbilical cord may prevent sensitization of some Rh- mothers, in some instances, against Rh+ blood. It is not, however, absolute prevention. Mothers with Rh- blood type should discuss this with their health provider and consider having mercury free Rhogam (short for Rh-immune globulin) following the birth of any Rh+ baby. A direct coombs test will give conclusive results concerning sensitization.

Even a short delay in clamping & cutting the cord makes a difference!

Two hundred seventy-six healthy women with uncomplicated pregnancies were randomized into three groups: cord clamping immediately after birth, at 1 minute and at 3 minutes. Venous hematocrit (to measure anemia) and bilirubin (to measure pathologic jaundice) were drawn at 6 hours and 24-48 hours after birth. Newborn physical exams were performed by clinicians who did not know to which group the infant was assigned.

Anemia at 6 hours of age was significantly more common in newborns who were randomized to the immediate cord clamping group. There was also a significant difference at 24-48 hours of age (16.8% of newborns in the immediate clamping group versus 2.2% at 1 minute and 3.3% at 3 minutes). Significantly more infants in the 3-minute group had elevated hematocrit levels (polycythemia) at 6 hours of age. However, none of the polycythemic babies exhibited symptoms or required treatment, and this difference did not persist to 24-48 hours of age. There were no significant differences in bilirubin values, rates of neonatal adverse events, or the infants' weight gain and rate of exclusive breastfeeding in the first month of life. There were no significant differences in maternal outcomes such as blood loss or maternal hematocrit levels.[13]

Cord Blood Banking

There has been much research conducted that questions the usefulness and ethics of umbilical cord blood banking. In addition to the issues already discussed with clamping and cutting the umbilical cord too early, I wonder if banking umbilical cord blood is virtually unnecessary if the full amount of cord blood and precious stem cells are allowed to flow into the baby at birth. Some have even found that denying babies their cord blood may have explicitly adverse affects on the child, leading to ill health.

Banking umbilical cord blood is preemptive science, and it may even be a solution that causes problems. Overall, I believe that there is not enough evidence supporting the usefulness of banking the cord blood above just allowing the baby his or her birthright of cord blood and stem cells to insure a strong immune response to potential future diseases. Preventing newborn anemia, by delaying the clamping and cutting of the umbilical cord, predisposes children to healthier lives and a reduced need for highly technological attempts at cures later in life.

Kelly Winder, professional doula and creator of the online parenting website *www.bellybelly.com.au*, lays the issue out most succinctly in her article *Why Delaying Cord Clamping Benefits Your Baby*:

> *"Umbilical cord blood is a baby's lifeblood until birth. It contains many wonderfully precious cells, like stem cells, red blood cells, and more recently scientists have discovered that umbilical cord blood contains cancer-fighting T-cells. Yet common practice is to cut this source of valuable cells off from the baby at the moment of birth, due to unsubstantiated claims that it can cause complications. Not only that, a new line of business has been set up to store this precious cord blood for you...Collection is also very lucrative for the collector (midwives get offered training in this too, some decline but some do it). Collectors get paid hundreds for doing the procedure."* [14]

How likely is it that a baby will need stored stem cells? According to Dr. Sarah Buckley, in her book *Gentle Birth, Gentle Mothering*, the likelihood of low-risk children needing their own stored cells is approximately 1 in 20,000. She also reveals that "Cord blood donations are likely to be ineffective for the treatment of adults, because the number of stem cells are too few." [15]

I suspect that my children, grandchildren and the other babies I receive into the world get their birthright of precious stem cells by leaving their cords intact and allowing the placental blood to enter their bodies. The businesses that collect and store umbilical cord blood make a good case for the value of this blood. How they justify robbing newborns of their cord blood at birth – remember, collecting cord blood requires the immediate clamping and cutting of the umbilical cord – is beyond my comprehension. The "Why?" is quite obvious: to make lots of money! I don't feel my babies missed out because their families chose not to pay steep fees to bank their umbilical cord blood, on the chance that future developments in medical science will make these artificially preserved stem cells useful in treating possible future cancers. The research proves immediate clamping and cutting of the cord causes newborn anemia, contributing to diminished health and perhaps even diminished intelligence. I prefer to gamble on nature, insuring that babies get their full blood supply at birth to prevent future illnesses.

Cruel experiments are carried out on living animals to monitor the safety of certain products before allowing their use for humans. Anti-vivisectionists have pointed out that there is evidence that the same experiments can be carried out on placentas, which respond to stimulus just as if they are alive, for the first five hours following birth. To me this further establishes the need for us to leave the baby, cord and placenta intact for many hours following birth. If the placenta behaves as a living being for up to five hours following birth, it must indeed still be functioning to assist the baby, just as it did in the womb.

Expectant parents have the right and responsibility to ensure that their babies can enjoy optimal lives. Cutting the umbilical cord is a violent procedure that is inherently dangerous. Leaving the cord intact, un-amputated, unclamped and uncut until the cord is no longer pulsing at all (even near the baby; this can take an hour or more, even three hours, in my experience) is essential if optimal health of the baby is to be achieved.

Hospitals are businesses, which means that they should listen to the wishes of their consumers. If you are planning a hospital birth, insist on your right to choose optimal health for your baby. For the most part midwives believe in and practice gentle birth. Planning a home or birth center birth attended by midwives makes the decision not to sever your baby's cord immediately an easy one. It is the decision I recommend for most mothers and babies. Let us help medical professionals, who are meant to protect health, do their job, by asking them to leave our babies umbilical cords intact, the obvious healthier choice.

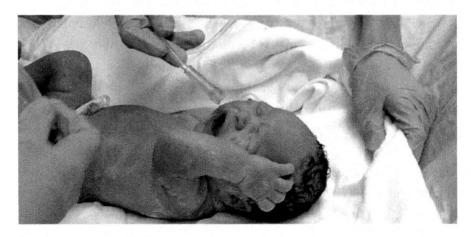

How about Premature Babies?

Should health providers delay the clamping and cutting of umbilical cords of premature babies?

Yes, delay the severance of premies from their umbilical cords/placentas, as long as possible. According to Kugelman et al in the *American Journal of Perinatilogy*, 2007, studying preterm neonates of less than 35 weeks gestation at the time of birth found: The investigators observed that the DCC (delayed cord clamping) group had initial higher diastolic BP and higher Hct values, but did not develop polycythemia. Low birth weight (<1500 grams) babies in the DCC group also required lesser surfactant and mechanical ventilation. The phototherapy needs of infants with higher bilirubin levels in the DCC group however remained at par with those in the ICC (immediate cord clamping) group.[16]

A Premature Baby's Story...

Julia's amniotic fluid had gushed out, all over the home of her friend Silvia, who was putting Julia and her two daughters up while the family awaited the return of Jason, Julia's husband, who was working in NYC. Julia had been putting in too many hours looking for the right home to rent. She was planning on a homebirth, just like the first two, and wanted everything to be ready when her husband arrived. Silvia felt Julia was pushing herself to exhaustion and becoming hungry and dehydrated, day after day, house hunting while the girls were in school. When Julia's waters released she cried, "I can't have this baby now, I'm only 33 weeks pregnant!"

Sylvia took Julia to the birth center where she had birthed a year earlier, feeling the midwives would know what to do. They arrived late at night. The midwives evaluated Julia, found her to be barely 33 weeks along, with definite premature rupture of membranes (PROM). They called their back-up OB doctor and she advised the midwives to let the exhausted mom sleep, as there were no contractions yet. In the morning labor began gently. The doctor and the midwives decided to allow Julia to labor slowly, and pray for a good outcome. At about dinnertime Julia got into the birth tub. Her husband was still on the plane from New York. Ever so gently, in the waterbirth tub Julia birthed her third baby, a boy. Aaron was small, but at 2.2 kg. he had good APGAR scores, so he would not need to be transferred to neonatal intensive care. Juila kept him skin-to-skin and intact with his placenta. Attempts to help Baby Aaron to the breasts failed, as he was just too weak and had no sucking reflex. The midwives fed Julia red rice cereal every two hours, as it was known to bring a mother's milk in faster, and there was research to prove it. Julia pumped her breasts often and by the end of the first day postpartum, she had a good 20cc of colostrum every few hours, to feed the baby via syringe.

Julia and her daughters decided to wait for Papa Jason to arrive on the island, before severing the baby's umbilical cord. He slept, woke, peed and pooped and most importantly, he breathed without trouble. When Baby's father finally arrived it was late on the 3rd day. He was surprised to see his premature baby doing so well. The next day they decided to burn the cord. Julia continued to pump and feed her baby breast milk, exclusively. In less than two weeks baby Aaron was 3.3 kilograms, he was exclusively breastfed and thoroughly loved by his family. Jason, the father, had been a little taken aback by the sight of his son, three days old, with the dried umbilical cord and salted placenta still attached. A few months later he told the midwives how he felt that the gentle vaginal birth, exclusive breastfeeding and skin-to-skin care, plus the placenta, all contributed to the baby's ability to thrive perfectly even though he was born seven weeks early.

According to Costa Rican midwife, Vanessa Calderon, the *parteras* (midwives) that she has known in Mexico, Panama and Costa Rica sit with the family members in quiet celebration after the baby's birth. They eat, drink tea and coffee and smoke cigarillios. Nearly all of the old women who deliver the babies smoke. This comes in handy when they wish to go home and, before doing so, want to finish up the birth. The *parteras* simply use the burning ember of the cigarillio they are smoking to cauterize and sever the umbilical cord.

Placentas and GMO Foods

Dear sister midwives, nurses, doctors, doulas and Birth Keepers, I am writing from Indonesia, the country who got GMO soy very early, to share what I am seeing, and ask if you too are seeing the same, and begin a dialog...

In 2008, Bumi Sehat Bali received 573 babies. We saw an increase in retained placentas. We often see hemorrhage, due to malnutrition; A big problem since the 1970s, when green revolution rice was introduced resulting in a profound impact on maternal mortality in Bali. Also, I am seeing an increase in velamentous cord insertion.*

One would expect, given the rate of malnourishment here, that the birthing women would use every bit of Qi to push out their babies, leaving little or not much Qi for releasing the placenta and involution. However, in 2008 and so far in 2009, we have seen too many 'sticky' placentas. (When absolutely necessary, we perform manual removal of retained placenta, but two of the women from this period required transport. One resulted in a hysterectomy, the other, in the hands of Dr. Wedagama, our backup surgeon, just avoided surgery but lost over 1 liter of blood. With usually no more than one manual removal per year, in the last 6 weeks of 2008, I had to manually remove 4 placentas! It was not pretty, and I do not take it lightly.)

Also, most shocking is my empirical experience (I have yet to find upporting research) of seeing an increase of velamentous umbilical cord insertion and short cords since the introduction of GMO foods to Indonesia.

Two weeks ago, Padma arrived at the birth center in labor with her 4th child. She had been vegetarian for 15 years, her third baby died the week before birth, from

---

* Normally, the cord inserts into the middle of the placenta. In velamentous cord insertion, the umbilical cord inserts into the membranes, then travels within the membranes to the placenta (between the amnion and chorion). The exposed vessels are not protected by Wharton's jelly and hence are vulnerable to rupture. Rupture is especially likely if the vessels are near the cervix, in which case they may rupture in early labor (causing a stillbirth).[17]

what was diagnosed as a cord accident. This 4th baby was born healthy, but the umbilical cord was flat, 4 to 5 cm wide (looked like a tape worm) and had five skinny vulnerable vessels arriving each separately to the placenta!!! The placenta was not the lovely placentas I know and love. There was no Wharton's jelly around the cord to speak of (with many babies I am seeing a decrease in Wharton's jelly). The placenta was very thin, 1 ½ to 2 cm in thickness. It covered a large area, spreading out far and wide (approx 30 cm diameter) across the top half of the uterus, with deep root-like 'feet' that I had to carefully tease off of the uterine wall. It's a miracle the baby did not break this very vulnerable cord, break it and die while still gestating. It's also a miracle this placenta could be manually removed, and that this mother survived. I am hoping she is not planning any more pregnancies.

Last week a young mom lost her baby in labor... suddenly FHT went from 150 to zero exactly 15 minutes between listening times... there was no dipping or drop in heart tones, just suddenly, absence of life. Five hours later, a lovely baby girl was born dead. There was no hope. The cord was less than 30 cm long and had been pulled too hard as it was wrapped tightly around her foot. This mom is very poor, her husband has no job, their only source of protein is tempe made from soy.

Recently, we had a 2nd time mom come in, very poor and malnourished. On arrival FHT were above 160, she was 9 cm, but nothing we did to try to stabilize the baby worked. As FHT reached 188 and continued to climb (that is with O2 support! and hands and knees), we transported... stat cesarean, baby very weak, low APGAR... but the baby came around and our staff midwife retreived her from the hospital nursery and he went straight onto the mother's breast. This baby would not have survived our normal hands-off gentle birth. Saved by O2, a doppler and cesarean. This the kind of drama that unfolds when the placenta is underdeveloped and the cord too short.

And the cords we are seeing are shorter. Last week emergency circumstances led to our midwife Ayu cutting a cord after the birth of the head, as the body would not follow; It was that short a nuchal cord!* She had never had to do this before in her life as a midwife!

---

* Nuchal cord occurs when the umbilical cord is wrapped around the fetal neck 360°.

These are just a few daring stories, but we are alsoseeing many less dramatic examples of shorter cords, velamentous cord insertion, diminished Wharton's jelly, and abnormal looking placentas.

Dita, having her second baby, was stuck at 9 cm (with a transient but strong intermittent urge to push) from 7 pm until the next morning at 8:30 when she finally got complete; After hands and knees with butt up, moxa kidney 1 (ball of foot), homeopathic pulsatilla to disengage baby from pelvis and then elephant walking stairs to bring him down right. We had had strange bleeding in first stage, but baby remained strong and stable and mom was quite well through the long labor. We were careful not to rush the labor, in case it was a short or nuchal cord; we wanted the cord to stretch gently. Twenty minutes before the birth, FHT were suddenly absent. Hands and knees, O2 and slowly, slowly, he came back. Dita felt a strong urge to get her baby out. He was most stable when she squatted, not our preferred gentle birth, we were in high risk territory. She had to push very hard now, as we had no time to transport. Dita did it, her son was born by her own power and all of our prayers to Allah (Dita is Muslim). Alhamdulillah! Our 3.6 kilo baby boy's cord was short, just about 40 cm, with velamentous insertion... AGAIN! Yet another abnormal umbilical cord. Dita's main source of protein is soy.

One week in August, 2010, we had five babies in a 12 hour night... two had velamentous cord insertions! It's just not average anymore. In five days time, I saw one fatal cord accident, another cord problem leading to stat cesarean birth, and another incident of deep fetal distress due to cord problems.

I am wondering what other Birth Keepers are seeing?

Can you see why I am worried about our precious placentas? I did not make this connection until I began to see an increase in abnormalities and pathology due to placenta and cord troubles. The fact that so many Indonesian women and their families depend upon genetically modified soy products (tempe and tofu) for their day-to-day protein has me wondering if there is a connection between the many abnormal placentas and short cords we are seeing in our vegetarian mothers. A vegetarian dependent upon GMO soy. I don't want to jump to conclusions, I only wish to ask the question: Is GMO soy contributing to abnormalities in placentas and umbilical cords? I HOPE this is not a trend or a pattern. We really don't want GMO foods or other factors, i.e. environmental pollutants, pesticides etc. to lead to abnormal changes in placentas. It would be a devastating man made tragedy.

As I prepare this manuscript for publication (August 2010), I was called in to help the midwives cope with a serious retained placenta and hemorrhage. After I was able, with difficulty, to manually remove the adhered placenta, I noticed it looked like many I had seen in vegetarian moms. I asked Ibu Wayan Rima, "Are you vegetarian?" Her answer was, "Yes." I explained that I had seen this problem in many vegetarian women and that I was concerned that there might be complications if even a tiny bit of the placenta which had been unnaturally rooted in her uterus, remained inside. I told Wayan that one way to prevent further complications was for her to eat a small piece of her placenta. Her husband, a Hindu priest encouraged her, "It's meat from birth, not death. I think it's good." He had seen how his wife suffered due to the manual extraction of her placenta, which had saved her life. He also feared further complications. Ibu Wayan ate one cotyledon of her placenta, coated in honey. A few hours later, her unexpected recovery amazed the midwives.

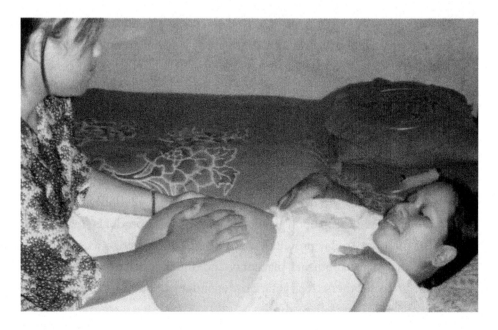

Some disturbing research concerning human umbilical, embryonic and placental cells:

> *"We have evaluated the toxicity of four glyphosate (G)-based herbicides in Roundup (R) formulations, from 10(S) times dilutions, on three different human cell types. This dilution level is far below agricultural recommendations and corresponds to low levels of residues in food or feed. The formulations have been compared to G alone and with its main metabolite AMPA or with one known adjuvant of R formulations, POEA. HUVEC primary neonate umbilical cord vein cells have been tested with 293 embryonic kidney and JEG3 placental cell lines. All R formulations cause total cell death within 24 h, through an inhibition of the mitochondrial succinate dehydrogenase activity, and necrosis, by release of cytosolic adenylate kinase measuring membrane damage. They also induce apoptosis via activation of enzymatic caspases 3/7 activity. This is confirmed by characteristic DNA fragmentation, nuclear shrinkage (pyknosis), and nuclear fragmentation (karyorrhexis), which is demonstrated by DAPI in apoptotic round cells. G provokes only apoptosis, and HUVEC are 100 times more sensitive overall at this level. The deleterious effects are not proportional to G concentrations but rather depend on the nature of the adjuvants. AMPA and POEA separately and synergistically damage cell membranes like R but at different concentrations. Their mixtures are generally even more harmful with G. In conclusion, the R adjuvants like POEA change human cell permeability and amplify toxicity induced already by G, through apoptosis and necrosis. The real threshold of G toxicity must take into account the presence of adjuvants but also G metabolism and time-amplified effects or bioaccumulation. This should be discussed when analyzing the in vivo toxic actions of R. This work clearly confirms that the adjuvants in Roundup formulations are not inert. Moreover, the proprietary mixtures available on the market could cause cell damage and even death around residual levels to be expected, especially in food and feed derived from R formulation-treated crops.*[18]

In 2005, Irina Ermakova, along with the Russian National Academy of Sciences, reported that more than half the babies from mother rats fed GM soy died within three weeks. This was five times higher than death rate of the non-GMO soy group. The babies in the GMO group were also smaller and could not reproduce.[19]

What About HIV/AIDS?

While reading the medical literature to see if delaying the clamping and cutting of the umbilical cord is counter indicated for HIV+ mothers, I found that the studies showed invasive obstetrical protocols should be avoided during the birth of a baby with an HIV+ mother.

> *"Other obstetrical modifications can reduce contact between the infant and the mother's infected body fluids. These involve avoiding episiotomies, unnecessary artificial rupture of membranes, fetal scalp electrodes and other invasive procedures."* [20]

In addition to the above list of obstetrical procedures to reduce the incidence of Mother-to-child transmission of HIV/AIDS, I would suggest the avoidance of multiple vaginal exams, especially after membranes have ruptured, fundal pressure during the pushing stage of labor, instrument delivery (i.e. forceps or vacuum extractor). Any trauma to the baby must be avoided, vigorous suctioning of the infant is not recommended as it causes trauma to baby's mucous membranes,[21] also avoid aggressive third stage delivery of the placenta. In other words, gentle birth is a researched based, sound model for prevention of HIV/AIDS transmission to babies. Reducing the rate of mother to child transmission of HIV virus was more dependant upon the mother getting antiretroviral drugs during pregnancy and labor than the timing of the umbilical cord severance.

> *"Among mothers with membranes that ruptured more than four hours before delivery, the rate of transmission of HIV-1 to the infants was 25 percent, as compared with 14 percent among mothers with membranes that ruptured four hours or less before delivery. In a multivariate analysis, the presence of ruptured membranes for more than four hours nearly doubled the risk of transmission (odds ratio, 1.82; 95 percent confidence interval, 1.10 to 3.00; P = 0.02), regardless of the mode of delivery. The other maternal factors independently associated with transmission were illicit-drug use during pregnancy (odds ratio, 1.90; 95 percent confidence interval, 1.14 to 3.16; P = 0.01), low antenatal CD4+ lymphocyte count (<29 percent of total lymphocytes) (odds ratio, 2.82; 1.67 to 4.76; P<0.001), and birth weight <2500 g (odds ratio, 1.86; 1.03 to 3.34; P = 0.04)."* [22]

Honoring the
Third Stage of Labor:
The Birth of the Placenta

A woman dies due to a complication of pregnancy or childbirth every minute of everyday, 365 days a year. Most of these deaths are due to hemorrhage in the third stage of labor, after the baby has been born, in the process of or shortly following the delivery of the placenta. This fact should be enough to convince birth keepers to hold the birth of the placenta as a physical and spiritual event of extreme importance. The trouble is that, once the baby is born, even very conscious midwives and doctors tend to handle the placenta's birth as merely a mechanical process. I believe that by holding the third stage of labor in the highest regard, remembering that it is driven by the mother's oxytocin, that very shy hormone of love, we would see fewer postpartum hemorrhages.

Before there were medications to stop hemorrhage, there were other methods used by traditional birth attendants. These midwife-witches - sage fem, *dukun bayi*, hilot, dais, grannies - trusted by their communities, still work today in the remote regions of the world to assist women in pregnancy, labor, childbirth, postpartum and the support of breastfeeding. Many of them have no access to anti-hemorrhagic drugs, nor do they have syringes and needles with which to administer injections. Many of them live far away from medical backup and serve the world's most marginalized, isolated, impoverished, malnourished, high-risk moms. Yet, they are able to use the simple knowledge passed down from their grandmothers, the bravery of their hearts, and the skill of their hands to stop life threatening hemorrhage.

Most traditional birth attendants know from experience that putting the baby to the breast immediately after birth is the best way to stimulate the safe delivery of the placenta. Separation of mother and baby puts the mother at greater risk for postpartum hemorrhage. Many of the traditional midwives use various plants as allies and herbal remedies, but herbs are often seasonal and they take time to prepare. When a mom begins to bleed, the midwife must be ready to use what she has on hand to reliably stop hemorrhage. For this, she may employ the placenta.

There are druid stories of the granny midwife saving the hemorrhaging mother by instructing her to suck on a corner of her placenta. In my practice in Bali and in Aceh, I could not imagine getting a woman, who is culturally afraid of and revolted by blood, to do this. Yet I serve a population of women who are predisposed historically and nutritionally to hemorrhage after giving birth. In Chinese medicine we would say that these women use up all of their Qi while giving birth. They are so wiped-out by hunger, malnutrition and exhaustion due to a hard life, that they don't have enough Qi to successfully complete the birth process: fully delivering the placenta and successfully clamping down the uterus to stop the bleeding.

In Bali, hemorrhage after childbirth is the leading cause of death.[1] Because so many of our birth mothers hemorrhage at Bumi Sehat Bali and Aceh, we keep anti-hemorrhagic medicines close at hand. Yunnan Baiyao, a patented, easy to find hemostatic powder (Chinese medicine, consisting of Tienchi ginseng and Rhizoma Dioscoreae) dissolved in warm water with a couple of tablespoons of honey, helps the mother deliver her placenta, reduces bleeding and encourages milk production. If the mom continues to bleed, we administer pitocin by injection. If that does not stop the hemorrhage, we give Methylergometrine by injection (provided the mom is not suffering from hypertension). Once the placenta is delivered, we check to make sure there are no missing cotyledon (bits of placenta), amnion or chorion left inside, which can cause her to hemorrhage dangerously. If she is still bleeding, we graduate to giving Misoprostol anally, which is an almost surefire remedy for stopping the hemorrhage. It is also long lasting, so it will continue helping the mother's uterus maintain integrity, often until her body has resolved the cause of the hemorrhage.

However, in my midwifery practice, there have been many times when these measures did not stop hemorrhage. I can recall a rather frightening November in 2007 when this happened four times in one month. I was faced with going into the woman's uterus to manually check for leftover bits of placenta, amnion, chorion and blood clots, or putting in an IV line and transporting the mom to the hospital for dilation and curettage (D&C) and blood transfusions. Delays in resolving the cause or hemorrhage or transport problems in the case of extreme hemorrhage can cost lives. In each situation, the mom was bleeding profoundly and medications would not stop the hemorrhage. I felt an urgent need to feed the bleeding mother a piece of her placenta.

I had to act fast. I put on a new pair of sterile gloves and reached for the placenta, which is always in a bowl beside the mom, still connected to the baby. I pinched off a tiny bit and asked my assistant midwife pour honey on it. We keep a bottle of honey on hand at all births and strongly suggest all midwives and OBGYN doctors do the same, as honey can dramatically revitalize a laboring mom during the second stage of labor while she is pushing. Next, I quickly scooped up the honey-coated bit of placenta and asked the mother, "May I ask you to swallow this real placenta medicine. It will help you." When she agreed, I popped it in her mouth and gave her a swig of water.

In each case, when none of the medications worked, the hemorrhaging stopped immediately within minutes of the mother ingesting a small bit of her own placenta. The mom's uterus became rock hard and she stopped bleeding out. In one case, it was not the uterus that would not clamp down, but the mother's cervix, which was incompetent. This mother, Reni, had required transfusions and nearly died of hemorrhage following her previous birth. However, after ingesting a small amount of her own placenta, Reni's cervix shut tight and she was saved; her blood pressure held stable and she did not need blood transfusions.

All four mothers had lost a significant amount of blood – 800ml to 1 liter, yet none of them suffered significant drops in blood pressure. Only one was put on IV fluids afterwards. None of the mother's who had hemorrhaged required blood transfusions. They were so well, in fact, that they needed no special postpartum care, except for observation, good nutritious foods and breastfeeding support. All of the mothers were pleased and proud of the fact that their placentas helped them.

I never would have expected my friend Ingrid, a tall Dutch woman married to a man from the island of Flores, to hemorrhage after the birth of her second baby. She arrived at the airport in Bali and her water released. She called to tell me she was beginning labor, though she thought she had three weeks more of pregnancy. I asked her to come quickly to the Bumi Sehat birth center. Almost immediately after she arrived, she was in the birth tub and soon after, her baby girl was in her arms. "Well, I made it to Bali," Ingrid beamed at the Baliniese midwives attending her. "I was so afraid of bleeding like I did after my first baby's birth." Unfortunately, as soon as she uttered those words, the birth tub turned a deep red. Her midwife Gung Sayang did not reach for oxytocin, as she knew from Ingrid's history that medication would not help. Instead Gung Sayang nipped off a generous piece of the placenta, which was floating in a bowl in the birth tub, coated it with honey and fed it to Ingrid. Ingrid was more than happy to eat placenta, as she was terrified of bleeding again. Shortly after eating a piece of her placenta, Ingrid's uterus contracted effectively and she stopped bleeding. Her milk came in easily and the baby championed at feeding on her breasts. I asked Bidan Chantia, who assisted Gung Sayang that day, "Why did you give her such a big piece of the placenta to eat?" Chantia replied, "Because she is such a tall, large woman!" This brought laughter to all of us, including Ingrid, who was grateful that her baby's placenta had saved her life.

The protocol of feeding new mothers a bit of their baby's placenta to stop postpartum hemorrhage, as I have described it here, has been taught to traditional birth attendants in Aceh: After the Tsunami, they had no other methods available to preserve maternal life. This method is also being taught now in Nepal, Tibet and India among traditional birth attendants working far from modern hospitals.

The Sacred Trinity

In many faiths throughout history, the Trinity is sacred. The ancient mother religions honored the three stages of female life: Maiden, Mother and Crone. The Christian religion blesses the Father, the Son and the Holy Spirit - three divine persons in one divine substance. The ancient Greeks revered the Graces: Aglaia, Thalia, and Euphrosyne, daughters of Zeus, known as the Charities. They were believed to personify and bestow charm, grace, and beauty.* Hindus worship Brahma the creator, Vishnu the protector and Shiva the destroyer. Their Hindu female counterparts are Lakshmi, Parvati and Kali. Perhaps the Trinity is so deeply ingrained in our consciousness because we humans begin life as a triad being: baby, cord and placenta, the trinity of our sacred roots.

The Magi saw the birth of the Christ Child foretold by a star in the heavens. Angels appeared to them with glad tidings. These three wise men traveled to Bethlehem bearing gifts of gold, frankincense and myrrh. It was tradition in these times when welcoming a new baby to bring gifts of fragrant, aromatic, anti-bacterial herbs, resins and plant gums … perhaps the precious frankincense and myrrh were used for the placenta of Baby Jesus.

An Indonesian child whose placenta, called *Ari-ari* or Kakak – which means older brother or sister, is buried in the earth beside the family home will feel most comfortable there and will most likely live his life nearby. Many families send the placenta of one of their children out to the ocean for it's final rest. This person will grow to be adventurous, and bring home riches from the seven seas. When a Balinese baby's cord stump falls away, her parents will put it in a *Ketipat Kukur* and place it on an altar called a *Kumaran*.

---

* The poet Hesiod who named the Graces in his Theogony: *"Then Eurynome, Ocean's fair daughter, bore to Zeus the three Graces, all fair-cheeked, Aglaia, Euphrosyne, and shapely Thalia; their alluring eyes glance from under their brows, and from their eyelids drips desire that unstrings the limbs."*

Placenta Trauma

Rebirthing and breath-work therapists (therapeutic method of helping people relive past events to understand and relieve trauma) report many cases of people remembering the cutting of their umbilical cord and experiencing placenta trauma. They recall a range of feelings, from a nagging sense of having lost something or someone, to disassociation, longing for a missing twin, even the feeling of having suffered an amputation. Many move through a terrible feeling of dread, felt most intensely in the naval area or pit of the belly.

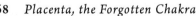

"The first time I encountered my 'placenta trauma' was during my very first rebirthing session, which happened to be about my birth. I saw something being thrown into a white enamel bucket and was not sure what it was. At the time I wondered if it was the placenta, but because I felt so close to it, and the pain of it landing in the bucket was so immense, I interpreted it to be a dead twin that was removed without mention. The bucket appeared many times in later sessions and each time caused the same amount of separation pain that stayed unresolved. I frequently considered whether the content could be the placenta, but discarded the thought/ feeling because I believed that the placenta was a part of the mother, after all in German it is called the Mutterkuchen (mother-cake). The intensity of feeling towards this 'being' in the bucket confirmed my belief that this must be more then an afterbirth, which in 1947 was not much more than a discardable leftover from the birth."

– Nemi Nath from *Wholly Whole: A Personal Case History of Placenta Trauma*

I believe that the placenta is truly alive, experiences emotions and has an intelligence of it's own. How do we explain why so may people live with feelings of being cut off from a significant part of themselves? Many of us experience a groundless fear, not exactly our own but infinitely related. Other people walk through life with a suspicion that they lost a twin at birth. The Hawaiians believe we are connected to people by *aka* cords (some are healthy connections and others not) and that many of us sense we have an *aka* cord that was violently severed and whips around wildly disrupting our lives. I can't help wondering if this severed cord is the umbilicus. Rebirthing experiences all over the world have confirmed that I am not alone in this wondering.

There are so many paths to wholeness. I have come to realize that, for most of us, becoming whole and truly functional is a process of naming the trauma of our birth and separation from placenta, accepting that pain as real and healing it by rejoining our fractured ethereal body. It is as if, at birth, we really did suffer "Original Sin" when our umbilical cord was quickly, harshly and, without warning, severed. We lost our identical twin, our doppelganger, our best friend, mirror image, brother or sister.

I grew up sensing that I had a very small, helpless sibling, who I was not able to protect. I searched for that sibling most of my life, even after my own children were born. This 'lost baby sister' haunted me. As a small child, I tried to replace the lost baby sister with a small toy panda bear named Nicky, who I carried around day and night. I held Nicky by a red ribbon tied around her neck and she was approximately the size of a placenta. Writing this book has been a beautiful process of healing that trauma, as I now understand that I am not alone in looking for my lost placental sister. Though I can never find her, I can nurture the baby I was when we were separated and forgive myself for not being able to protect her.

Many mothers are unaware of the trauma they experience when they give birth in a conventional setting where the cord is immediately clamped and cut. Many do not sense their baby's and placenta's pain, but most mothers feel repulsed when they see the cord cut. When the doctor allows the baby's father to cut the cord, what kind of message is that for the new mother and for the baby? I do not recommend that new fathers cut their baby's cord. This act casts the father in the role of 'separator' and may have a profound affect on the family dynamics.

In 1982, at a *Healing Death and Dying* workshop, I heard Dr. Elizabeth Kubler Ross say, "People are 100% repairable." I suggest we begin our own repair by healing the primal wound, the severing of our umbilical cord which separated us from our placenta, quickly followed by separation from mother. I believe that a newborn interprets this separation as abandonment and loss of her experiential universe. When we heal this first cut, our ethereal bodies will again be whole and all other healing will come more naturally and easily. I believe that my midwifery practice is a calling and a healing. For each baby and placenta I protect and keep intact prevents trauma and heals this world, one baby at a time.

According to the research outlined in Michel Odent's book, *The Scientification of Love*, birth trauma results in an impaired ability to love and is the origin of dysfunctional living. Damaged people can be unkind and unconscious. Whole people with an intact ability and capacity to love are the warp and weft of a functional society, the foundation of peace. If we are to heal the Earth before we lose our only home, we must protect and respect the start-up conditions of each and every individual human. So we, as people, can live simply and beautifully together and welcome an enlightened age of healing and vision on this beautiful planet. This watery planet, salty as tears and salty as the amniotic fluid we, every one of us, grew in.

By preserving the integrity of the placenta at birth (only possible by the slow transition of allowing the placenta to separate from the baby naturally, or without severing the umbilical cord too quickly), we keep the circular flow of energy within our individual bodies. The placenta connects all of our charkas, enabling us to live as integrated, whole human beings, curved around the circular flow of energy, oscillating in a yin-yang pattern. Also, because the placenta connects each of us to our mother, it is the placenta chakra that gives continuity to the generations. Each Earthly child connected to each and every mother are like nesting Russian Matryoshka dolls reaching forward and backward in time, forever. By keeping this continuity intact, we preserve our relationship with past, present and future.

Lost Placentas

Many of us lost our placentas. I was born in a military hospital and my parents were never consulted about the disposal of my placenta. You may have recently had a baby, and it never occurred to you before now to take home and honor your baby's placenta. Please, no regrets. The best thing about the past is that it can be healed. I wrote my placenta a letter, asking her for forgiveness. As a child my mother taught me to talk to my Guardian Angel to ask her for help and guidance, and I know that my placenta was listening.

Dear Placenta/my Angel,

Forgive me for being a small baby and not having the power to make a proper ritual to honor your body, which died at my birth. I trust that you are with me in spirit, protecting, guiding me. Thank you for blessing my life. Thank you for being a witness to my joys and sorrows. May my life be an example of service and peace.

In Love,
Robin

I encourage you to write your own little letter to placenta. It feels amazing. What do you have to lose, except a few regrets? You will never 'find' your lost placenta, however, remembering is healing. After writing this letter to my placenta, I burned it in the garden, in a circle of flowers. I imagined the smoke carrying my prayers, hopes, and dreams into the spirit world, where my placenta awaits me.

We live in a world of "mine", a world where we rely on mountains of possessions. I wonder if the roots of consumerism are planted in the practice of taking babies' cord and placenta away before they naturally let go. Trauma from being forced to let-go too quickly leads to the feeling of separation and abandonment, which can result in behaviors of grasping and even hoarding in extreme cases. For most of us, it is just an aching for someone lost who we cannot identify. It may be just a feeling of homesickness or the worry that a family member is missing. For me, it was a childhood obsession with a stuffed panda bear about the size of my lost placenta that I affectionately named Nicky. I carried Nicky around under my right arm until it fell apart. Many times my mother repaired the damage and when he needed to be washed, I cried and stood beside the washing machine and dryer until he came out.

Then and even now, I feel the loss in my belly, right where my umbilical cord once attached me to my placenta.

In 2007, I was asked to speak at the 22nd Congress of Non-violence in Verona, Italy, about gentle birth as a foundation for peace on earth. Before commencing my speech, I led the audience in a brief experiment. I asked them to stand up and take hold of their purse or bag. Next I picked up my own bag, put the strap to my belly and asked all present to do the same. I then instructed the audience to take a moment of silence and focus on connecting to our center chakras and the bag we each held. Then I dropped my bag to the floor and instructed the audience to do the same. When they did I said, "Now imagine you have lost this bag forever." Immediately, a man in the audience exclaimed, "Oh! If I loose this bag I will die." His bag was round and red-brown, the strap was long, and I thought it resembled a placenta and cord. When other members of the audience shared similar feelings of panic for losing their bag, I asked them where they felt the loss in their body. They pointed to their gut right over their belly button, where their umbilical cord was once attached. I said, "Now what happened there when you were born?" It was then that they understood: the severing of their umbilical cord and placenta from their body left a lasting scar of separation and fear of loss.

Considered the deceased twin of the Ibo child in Nigeria and Ghana, the placenta is given full rituals for the dead and a burial.

How to Keep Placenta and Placenta Ceremonies

The easiest way to keep your placenta is to have a homebirth. However, I recommend discussing your plans before deciding on a midwife to confirm that she will respect and carry out your wishes. You should be specific: tell her whether or not you want the cord cut. If you do not want it cut (as in a Lotus Birth, discussed further in the next chapter), then you should share with her your specific wishes for how you want the placenta to be handled. If you do want to have the cord cut, let her know at what point you want it cut and the method you want used: cutting or burning

If you are planning to have your baby in a birth center or hospital, you may face challenges or obstructions as to how you want your placenta to be handled. There may be laws, which vary by state and county, governing birth procedures, that could stand in your way. Hospitals often follow certain protocol concerning what they consider "medical waste" and do not want to be flexible. However, if you plan ahead, there is a chance that you can arrange for some or all of your wishes for your placenta to be carried out. Speak with your primary health care provider, doctor or midwife, whoever will be receiving your baby. Let them know you are serious and may change birth plans, including finding a new health provider and birth facility, if you cannot take home your placenta.

Make sure that the entire birth team – maternity nurses, attending midwives, doctors, etc - know about your plans for taking home your placenta. Remember, your partner will be busy bonding with his baby and falling more deeply in love with you. He should not be overly burdened with the task of protecting the placenta. A Doula (a person, usually a woman, who is professionally trained to assist a woman during childbirth and who may provide support to the family after the baby is born), who is trained to go with you to birth and protect you in the blessed labor, birth and postpartum process, is often the perfect person to guard the placenta. An understanding maternity nurse can also help you out. Again, plan ahead: when you pack your bag for the hospital, include two (good idea to double bag) heavy-duty Ziplock freezer bags, or a two-quart plastic bowl with a tight fitting leak-proof lid.

You have a right to keep your baby's placenta and create a meaningful ritual for laying it to rest. If even a tiny part of you believes, as people in many cultures believe, that the placenta is the physical body of the child's Guardian Angel, you must take it home.

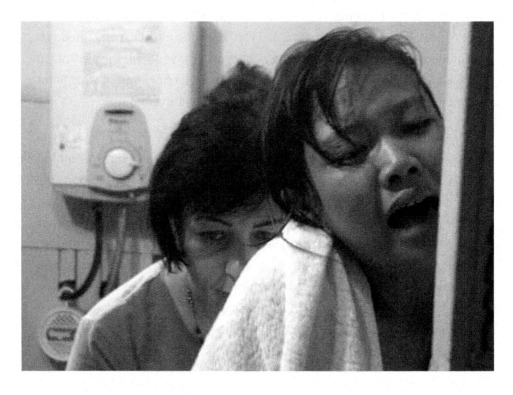

Placenta Take Home Check List

√ Agreement from hospital and health providers that you may take home your placenta

√ Two quart plastic bowl with tight fitting lid and/or two large, heavy-duty Ziplock bags

√ Partner, Doula or family member who will be at birth and ensure your wishes for your placenta are carried out

Pre-Birth Planning for Placenta Ceremony

These are just some of many options for your placenta ceremony. You may choose to create any kind of ceremony you want.

√ Buy a tree to plant and bury your placenta under

√ Write a letter of wishes to include in the burial site

√ Decide where the placenta will have its final rest

√ Bury in the ground either directly or in a pot, so it is portable and can be moved, if necessary

√ Take it far out to sea and "put her to rest" in the ocean

√ Bury placenta in the forest or where the baby was conceived

√ Decide who will be present to bless the placenta to rest

√ Spices for Pãté

Options for Parents to Consider When Planning Baby and Placenta's Birth

As parents-to-be, you have a once in a lifetime opportunity to plan for how your baby will be separated from his or her placenta. Just as birth is necessarily a parting between mother and baby, the placenta and baby will also be parted. The goal of this book is to minimize the separation trauma by helping families and healthcare providers execute it as gently as possible. Just as it is a well known fact that the best place for a newborn is right up on mother's belly, I propose that the best place for the placenta and baby is right beside each other while still connected by the umbilical cord for as long as possible. Remember, cord cutting needs to be a sterile procedure that requires the application of chemicals such as alcohol or Betadine, because it comes with some risks of infection. This is why it is done either by the doctor or midwife, or the baby's father, supervised by the healthcare provider. Again, I wonder about the message the baby receives when the father is the person who severs the cord?

The following are the options available to you as parents. Remember to choose what is the gentlest path that feels right for your family and the sweetest way you can imagine; your baby cannot choose, but depends upon you to be wise.

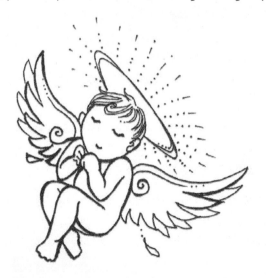

1. Immediate Clamping and Cutting of the Umbilical Cord

This is the medical model as done in most hospitals and birth centers in the world today. It has the advantage of being "easy", in that the parents need not say a thing or advocate at all. The doctor or midwife will simply clamp and cut the cord immediately after the baby is born, without discussion. Usually a plastic cord clamp is used, and this hard piece of plastic 3 to 4 cm in length does get between mother and baby when they are trying to initiate breastfeeding. Honestly, the clamp does cause the baby discomfort. If twisted or jammed into baby's belly, it causes pain. I advise that if you allow baby's cord to be cut, you ask for umbilical cord string or tape to be used instead of a clamp. Umbilical cord clamps look like small plastic monsters with teeth.

2. Delayed Clamping and Cutting of the Umbilical Cord

This is not too difficult to get your health provider to agree to. Advantages shown in the research are many, and only a 3 minute delay in umbilical cord clamping has many benefits for the baby. However, this and the first option mean that the cord will be cut before the birth of the placenta. This is very sad, in my opinion. Also, usually, a cord clamp will be used.

3. Prolonged Delay of Umbilical Cord Severance

This method is practiced by most midwives who receive babies at home and in more liberal childbirth centers and hospitals. These practitioners usually wait for about 15 minutes before clamping and cutting the cord. Sometimes this means the cord is severed before the placenta is even born. I strongly suggest that the parents ask the healthcare provider to wait at least until the placenta has been born. Even better is to wait until the baby has had its initial feed at the breast. After this, I believe the baby has gotten 99% of the physical benefits of delayed umbilical cord severance. Whenever we see the placenta, cord and baby (root, stem and fruit) intact, I call this a Lotus Birth.

4. Burning the Umbilical Cord

This method can be done after the placenta has been born and the baby has fed well at the breast. It cauterizes the umbilical cord, preventing infection and there is no need to use an uncomfortable cord clamp. According to traditional Asian medicinal knowledge, the burning of the umbilical cord moves the Qi (life force) remaining in the placenta into the baby. One slight disadvantage is that it takes 10 to 15 minutes to do, whereas cutting takes but a moment. Instructions for safely burning the umbilical cord are on page 46.

5. Waiting, Taking It One Day At A Time

Many families are not sure they wish to sever the cord immediately and have not decided on the method they are most comfortable with. I feel there is absolutely no hurry to decide. Leave the umbilical cord intact and review it as a family, one-hour or one day at a time. If you feel the transition time for baby is complete, you can always burn the cord after half a day, or one or two or three days following the birth. If the cord becomes brittle and breaks off before it releases at the bellybutton, don't distress, the baby must have been ready.

6. Full Lotus Birth

This is the most patient, spiritual, special way. To allow the cord to release from the baby with no rush, nothing but patience and non-violence. It is not for everyone, but it is worth the trouble. Families must be more mindful and move more slowly when handing the baby who is left intact with his or her umbilical cord and placenta. Although the baby who has had a few hours with her placenta has already gotten 99% or more of the benefits of delayed cord severance, I love Lotus Birth and feel it is the best possible start we can give our babies and grandbabies.

Placenta Prints

Some families that I have helped in homebirths have decided to honor the baby's placenta by making a print of it. This is quite easy to do. Just use a nice big piece of art paper. The blood serves as the ink. I simply pat it a bit, not too dry, and carefully place it on the print paper. First the baby's side, then the mother's side down. After the print has dried well, spray a bit of art fixative or regular old hairspray over the print. Let it dry again and frame.

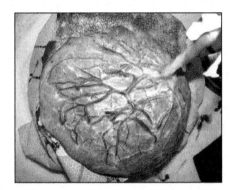 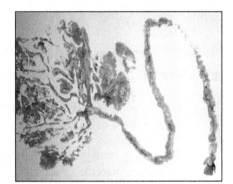

Indonesian families bury the baby's placenta with paintbrushes to bring artistic talent to the child. The mother who dreams her offspring will be a writer buries a pen along with the placenta. For a sweet disposition bury a sweet. A pinch of rice brings prosperity to the child's life ahead. In Bali a prayer written in Sanskrit which will bring spiritual wealth.

In New Zealand the placenta is buried in native soil. The Maori word for land, *Whenua*, is the same word for placenta. Quecha and Aymara fathers in Bolivia must bury their children's placentas in secret and always in the shade. Because these indigenous people believe that harm, even death, may come to mother and child if the ritual is not properly carried out, the placenta is treated with solemn respect.

Making a Dream Catcher

Asubakacin Bwaajige Ngwaagan:
Ojibwe language meaning "looks like a net dream snare"

A beautiful way to save and use the umbilical cord, which was the conduit delivering life to the baby, is to make a dream catcher. This tradition is said have its roots in Ojibwe and Chippewa Native American history. It is easy to do, and will be a delight to have. And, just maybe, it will filter out bad dreams while inspiring good.

There are several ways in which the umbilical cord may have been released from your baby and may be retrieved to make a dream catcher:

- If the cord was cut at the time of birth, either at home or in the hospital, ask your midwife or doctor to give you the cord.

- It may have been burned off. In this case ask for the umbilical cord and sever it from the placenta side in a respectful way.

- If your baby was Lotus born, meaning the cord was never cut or cut after some hours or days, respectfully sever it from the placenta before making the burial ritual for the placenta. In the case of Lotus Birth, you may wish to soak the cord in room temperature water for a while, until it rehydrates and becomes soft enough to form into the shape you choose. Or, it may be just the right leather like texture to go ahead and weave into a circle twisted upon itself.

In a bowl of water, wash the cord and gently push any blood inside of it out. It is not necessary to remove all of the blood, some dark spots will remain inside. If you have a Lotus Birth, removing blood may not be possible nor is it necessary.

Pat the umbilical cord dry. On a plate, arrange it in the shape you like: circle, spiral, heart, teardrop or infinity symbol, are some of a few we have done. Place the plate with cord in a dry place, away from family pets (they think it's a lovely chew toy!): on top of the refridgerator, the fireplace mantle, the television set (this is warm and makes it dry more quickly) or on top of the piano, all are good choices. Inside the oven has been found to be an unwise choice; if someone turns on the oven, the cord can quickly be burnt to ash.

Once the umbilical cord is dry, it will have shrunken quite a lot. You can pop it off of the plate by working a knife or your fingernail under a bit of it and gently moving or lifting. You may choose to store it in a nice medicine bag just as it is, or, you can bead any designs into and around it, making a string of beads to hang it up above and near where the baby will sleep. Traditionally, a web of string or sinew was woven into a spider's web pattern in the center to snare nightmares, while a small hole was left in the center to allow good dreams and wishes to come through and to be woven into the fabric of life. In the morning the nightmares would dissolve, just as the dew vanishes from the spider's web at the warming of the dawn. Feathers, symbols of breath, and beads of beauty were hung from the bottom of the dream catcher.

In the case of twins, I made two interlocking circles and beaded spider web like patterns in the centers of the cord circles. When I hung them up, I dangled carved whale and dolphin beads from the cord of baby Ocean, and a carved moon bead from baby Luna's cord. I hung them from one string, also decorated with beads.

In Turtle Island (North America), the people of the great lakes region would hang the dream catcher from the baby's cradleboard. If the umbilical cord was not saved, a dream catcher could be made with a supple willow branch and fiber or sinew string. Just as *Asibikaashi*, the Spider Woman, cared for her children of the land, the Placenta Spider Woman cares for each child as s/he journeys to Earth, from darkness into the light. The web of the dream catcher symbolizes her protection.

A Conversation Between Placenta and Child

By Joel Garnier

"Hey, I'm the placenta, ok?" "Ok." "Oops, mom's water just broke, don't panic." "Ok." "Soon we are going out there, ok, and you are going to have to learn to breathe air right away." "Ok". "Just sort of be as slippery and calm as you can, and I'll be right behind you." "I'm ready." "That's the spirit!" "Good pun!" "Nice work, you've got your head out. I've heard that's a trip, now relax one of your shoulders and you should glide right out." "Ok, I'm out. There are people here. What now?" "You've gotta blow your nose and clear your throat and start breathing air. I'll be out soon." "Someone just rested me in the crook of mom's arm, I'm breathing, I think it's safe to come out, hey, that thing you said about breasts, you were right. awesome!" "Ok, I'm out too, and these are good people, I'm over here in a bowl of flowers, still connected to you by our umbilical cord. I suggest you and mom catch some zeds and I'll be here when you wake up." "Cool" "Ok, it's morning, so wake up sleepy head." "Yeah, i've been awake, sort of." "Good, how is the air?" "It's nice. Yeah, really fresh, good smells." "Perfect, that is a really good sign." "Now what?" "ah, this is the part where we wait and see what they decide to do, you know, the parents. Don't take this the wrong way, but there's going to be some baby talk and a whole bunch of babbling and laughing that you and I won't understand. You might see some things, wait, I can't believe I forgot, did you open your eyes yet?" "Yeah, I told you I saw the breasts." "Right, right, sorry, say, have you, you know, suckled?" "Yep. and let me tell you sister, this is the best." "Ok, I'm a little jealous but I have all I need for the time being." "You know, I noticed the babbling and laughing and crying. What are they going on about?" "Who knows, it's always different." "You know, the cord is starting to dry up. Don't get all weepy on me." "Yeah, I know. I noticed that too. At least we get to stay connected for awhile longer." "Yeah. go to sleep. When you wake up I won't be here anymore. I can tell by what we've seen so far that you and mom are going to be fine and I'll be fine too, and if you listen carefully, you'll see that I have not really left you, ok?" "Ok, goodnight, I love you." "I love you too. Sweet dreams."

Lotus Birth

I would like to give special thanks to Brenda Richmond for her ideas and common sense. Brenda and her husband Meng have had two full Lotus born babies. Also huge thanks to my Daughter-in-love, Wine, and my son Noel, for deciding to give my grandson Bodhi Padma a full Lotus Birth. Of the thousands of families I have looked after as a midwife,* many have chosen Lotus Birth, in fact the numbers are increasing. Since 1999 I have done 10 to 12 full Lotus Births per year. All of the babies I receive have the benefit of having their placentas born and are breastfeeding before any thought of cord severance comes up. I believe that choosing when and if a baby's umbilical cord is to be severed, is a human right for all families.

I was a teenager the first time I saw a newborn baby intact with her umbilical cord and placenta, and the beauty of that sight took my breath away. Only an hour earlier I had become a mom. I was happily bonding with my new baby, Déjà, when my midwives asked me to squat over a bowl to release the placenta. They were feeling nervous, as more than an hour had passed since the birth of my baby, and the placenta was not yet born. I was not hemorrhaging, so there was no real hurry, but Mary and Debby felt our placenta was just sitting in my vagina, and it was time to release it. So I got up, holding my baby in my arms, still connected by our umbilical cord, and I squatted. When it came, I got to see the trinity of placenta, cord and my baby – the root, the stem and the fruit – as one. It was astonishing!

---

* To say thousands is not an exaggeration, I have been blessed to be a gentle birth midwife in a very busy place!

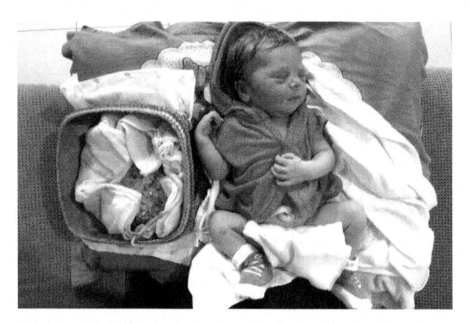

Just that: the placenta, umbilical cord and baby, born and still intact, is a Lotus Birth, according to the late June Whiston, who was my midwifery teacher and mentor. After that, the benefits are mostly spiritual and cannot be measured scientifically. A journey in gentle patience. Leaving the baby, cord and placenta intact until the cord dries and releases completely on its own, is a "full" Lotus Birth.

OK, leaving umbilical cords intact until they fall off naturally, which can take between 3 to 9 days, is way left of center to what has become considered normal on earth. However, historically humans did not always rush to sever the umbilical cord. If you consider the physical and spiritual benefits of leaving the cord and placenta attached to the baby, what is the basis for modern cultures' rush to separate the baby from her placenta?

I like to compare Lotus Birth to the slow process of growing a bonsai tree. It is all about patience – though a Bonsai tree takes years to craft and a Lotus Birth only takes days. Yet the ritual patience is the same. It requires the mother, baby and placenta to practice laying-in after childbirth in a trinity and spiritual bubble of transition. This allows, mother, baby and placenta the time and space to let-go gracefully, and only when they are truly ready.

There are many empirical experiences demonstrating that the longer you wait to cut the umbilical cord, the more physical and spiritual benefits the mother and baby feel and receive. In fact, the stem cells in umbilical cords are considered so valuable that cord blood banking companies charge families many thousands of dollars to save their baby's cord blood to use for potential future ailments. To me this does not make sense. Why would you want to save the precious stem cells for later when you can give your child the strongest possible entrance into the world by allowing them to migrate to the baby at birth.

Many still question the purpose of waiting for the cord to release by itself. Isn't it a hassle? Doesn't it stink? Waiting to cut the umbilical cord does take more intention and attention, but no, it does not need to stink if it is handled properly. And the purpose is simple: waiting a long time before severing the umbilical cord allows for the largest amount of nutrients and essential blood to enter the baby's body, protects the baby from suffering a violent physical act of detachment from his or her placenta and encourages immediate bonding with his/her mother. Leaving the cord attached to baby until it naturally falls off offers the baby and the family a rare opportunity to maintain a sacred space of patience and non-violence. Until one experiences a full Lotus Birth, it is nearly impossible to appreciate this sublime tender gentle way of introducing a new baby into the world.

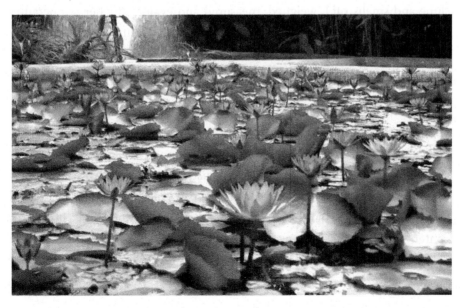

A close bond between mother and child is infinitely important and, in my experience, Lotus Birth facilitates that bond. While waiting for the umbilical cord to detach, the mother must lie close to the baby and placenta, breastfeeding in this sacred circle of quiet, restful seclusion; What midwives call "Baby-Mooning." Often, visitors don't feel as welcome while the placenta is still attached, so it is during this time that the family may bask in their own special glow as they are reinvented with the addition of the new baby.

What birthing women and their babies experience in most hospital settings (not only in the U.S., but everywhere, as western medicine has exported its protocols to developing countries), are procedures and practices that do not have intimacy and gentleness as a foundation. Once a woman in a hospital has reached full dilation, the vagina is made the enemy. With or without expulsion contractions (which only happen if the hormone oxytocin is allowed to do its job of kicking in the second stage of labor) women are told, and at times forced, to push. If she does not bring the baby out quickly enough, fundal pressure may be applied. Next, forceps or vacuum suction may be used. PUSH! PUSH! Episiotomies are cut to widen the birth canal and hasten the exit of baby, accomplishing the "rescue" in less time. Once born, the cord is immediately clamped and cut and the baby is immediately taken away from the mother. The baby is washed (getting all the "enemy" slime and smells off), weighed, measured and evaluated - her temperature taken anally. Finally, she is dressed and placed in a warmer – still kept away from her mother. Separation of baby from mother has become the normal routine in many many medical birth settings.

Even when birth becomes an emergency, as in depressed fetal heart rate or emergency cesarean, there is almost never a valid reason to immediately clamp and cut the baby's umbilical cord. The midwives and I in Bali have proven this many times. I was once criticized by an Australian sister midwife, as she saw the Bali midwifery team force a mother to push brutally to get her distressed baby born quickly. "That should have been done in a hospital, not a little birth center." The fact was, there was no time for transport. Once born, the baby was greeted with complete tenderness and left intact with his umbilical cord while we did CPR. This baby was revived right beside his mother, with her stroking him as we breathed for him and administered oxygen. All the while, he had the benefit of the placenta delivering help via the umbilical cord. When I see him at play in the village, I am certain that this was a gentle birth, a good birth.

Birth in most medical settings are a sharp contrast to the home births of my own children and grandchildren, and the births of the thousands of babies I've had the honor of receiving in their homes and at the Bumi Sehat birth center. Homes with extravagant carpets, homes with bamboo walls and packed mud floors, all those loving homes where birth took place without violence. The mother and baby were never kept apart in these homes. There were no high-tech infant warmers. The babies were warmed on their mother's skin, snug in her arms and cradled on her soft belly as they suckled at her breasts.

How to Have a Lotus Birth:
The Nitty-Gritty Details

As parents-to-be, you have a once in a lifetime opportunity to plan for how your baby will be separated from his or her placenta. As a midwife, I seek to minimize the separation trauma by helping families and health-providers execute the Lotus Birth as gently as possible. Just as it is a well known fact that the best place for a newborn is right up on mother's belly, I propose that the best place for the placenta is right beside the baby, still connected by the umbilical cord. Also, the best for baby is to be at mother's breasts, with placenta and papa as nearby as possible. Add a grandmother or two, and the recipe for landing on earth with the minimum of trauma is complete.

After the birth of the baby and the placenta, there is nothing to do except wrap the placenta in a towel and tuck it beside the mom and baby while they have their first breastfeeding adventure. Sometimes it is wise to put something like a chux pad or barrier between placenta and bedding to avoid blood and moisture wicking out onto the bed. Be mindful as you do this, so as not to pull the baby's cord when moving her around.

Next, the midwife or family member may bring a bowl of water to the bed and wash the blood away from the placenta. If you had a water birth, they can wash the placenta right there in the tub. Once the blood is thoroughly washed from the placenta, pat it dry and place it spongy side up (aka: the mommy side) on a dry towel. Salt it generously, making sure the salt is in all of the folds of the cotyledons. Now lay the placenta, mommy side down, in a small basket lined with a clean, dry cloth diaper or towel. A basket is better than a bowl, as it allows the placenta to breathe, preventing odor (washing and salting the placenta prevents odor too). Add more salt to the lovely shiny baby's side of the placenta and tuck this little package beside the baby. Make sure to change the placenta diaper every few hours, as it will absorb moisture from the placenta.

Some families express concern that the new grandparents would be upset by the presence of the umbilical cord and placenta still attached to the new grandbaby. In actuality, the grandparents of each Lotus Birth family I have known have been very supportive and pleased with the decision. None of them showed revulsion, nor did they criticize the parents for choosing this most gentle way.

Your family may wish to add some fragrant dry ground herbs to the salt sprinkled on your placenta. I use nutmeg most often, as it is easily available in Indonesia, where I live. I have also added dried rosemary, Indian chai herbs (cinnamon, clove, cardamom, ginger), and dried ground lavender flowers.

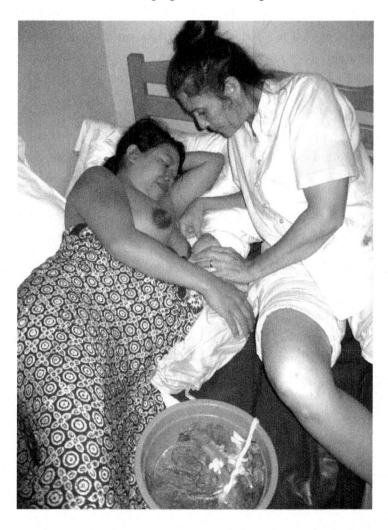

Lotus Birth After Cesarean

"Let's be realistic; let's do the impossible." ~ Che Guevara

If you need to have a cesarean birth, you can still enjoy a Lotus Birth. Cesarean Lotus Birth is rare, but it can be done. In Bali I work with three surgeons who will leave my patients' umbilical cords intact, even if the birth is by cesarean surgery. It is a blessing to have close, respectful, understanding relations with surgeons and doctors of obstetrics, for they can help facilitate the desires of birthing mothers, even when surgical birth becomes necessary. It is possible to have this type of relationship in other parts of the world too, if midwives and parents are willing to gently assert their desire for a Lotus Birth. Some doctors and surgeons may help, even in western countries where Lotus Birth is less common - you just need to try! I have now looked after more than a dozen mothers who needed cesarean birth and also chose Lotus Birth.

We were rushing the mother into surgery the first time I asked Dr. Hariyasa, a Balinese doctor of obstetrics, to leave the umbilical cord uncut for a mother I had transported to his hospital for an emergency cesarean. He looked at me and said, "Are you crazy?" as we were rushing the mother into surgery.

"You know I'm crazy!" I replied. He laughed and agreed, "Well, I guess now the hospital and the Department of Health will say I am crazy too!"

As the birth by surgery began, I softly sang the Gayatri mantra, a Hindu song of greeting for the human soul. The mother, who had spinal anesthesia and was awake, also sang, as did Dr. Hariyasa and Dr. Dharma, the anesthetist. Soon, I had to dab Dr. Hariyasa's eyes, as the song made him weep.

A few months later, Dr. Hariyasa's own daughter was born, and he and his wife also decided to have a Lotus Birth. It was then that I realized: Gentle birth really has a chance in this world if more Doctors refuse to cut their own children's umbilical cords.

Cesarean Lotus Birth of Chiyo & Liang

"In cases of caesarean section a higher incidence of respiratory distress occurs if placental transfusion does not take place. In-utero placental transfusion occurs if the fetus is hypoxic obviously to increase the oxygen supply to the fetal tissue. In conclusion: In order to give the newborn the blood, that it needs physiologically, cord clamping should be performed not immediately after birth, but one should wait as long until the umbilical vein has been empty and is collapsed." [1]

Chiaki of Japan and Gerry of Singapore came to me when they were expecting their first child. They wished for a completely non-violent beginning for their baby, so they chose to have a Lotus Birth.

While Chiaki was pushing, the baby's heart rate fell to 30 beats per minute. I put her on her hands and knees and gave her oxygen. The baby's heart rate increased, but with each push it decelerated again dangerously. It was time to move to the hospital. Chiaki and Gerry were broken hearted, as they had wished for their baby to have a Lotus Birth, and they thought this was not possible if she gave birth in the hospital.

As we wheeled Chiaki into surgery, I quickly negotiated with the hospital director, our surgeon and the pediatrician on-call, and they agreed to allow a lotus cesarean birth.

As Dr. Ardika made the first cut, the team sang the Gayatri mantra of healing. Although baby Chiyo was in deep distress, they didn't cut her umbilical cord. We rushed her to the resuscitation table and gave oxygen while I breathed for her. Slowly she came into her blue body and, finally, breathed a tiny cry. Yet her muscle tone was still weak and her blood sugar was low, so the pediatrician wished to give the baby some glucose via IV. I suggested we administer the glucose through the still-intact umbilical cord. As soon as we did this, Chiyo pinked up and made a hearty cry. Forty-three minutes later, baby Chiyo, still intact with her cord and placenta, was drinking from her mother's breast.

Gerry, Chiaki and Chiyo left the hospital 3 days later with their baby attached to her placenta. They named the placenta "Liang", which means lotus.

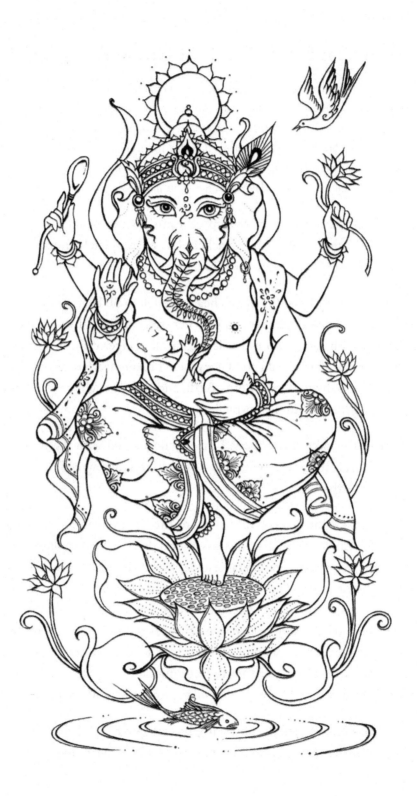

Lotus Birth Stories

"Once we had the placenta wrapped up and secure, it was fine. It was a small bundle to carry with the child. Because you already need to be gentle carrying the baby, it's not a big deal to have to be gentle when carrying the placenta. It felt good to be as soft as possible with the newborns - no cutting or ripping. Peaceful beginnings are good beginnings indeed."

– Sammy Shapiro, two-time Lotus Birth Dad

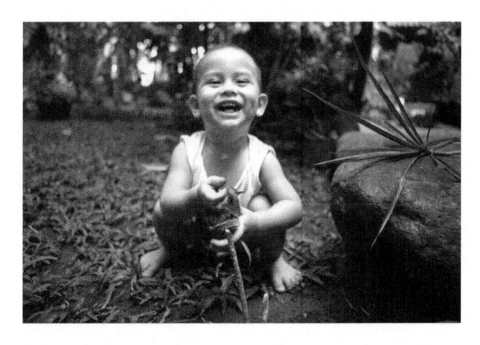

Bake The Cake

by Elena Skoko, excerpt from her Memories of a Singing Birth

"Oh, baby, you make me feel so good
Your rhythm just got my blues
This feeling is like a strawberry shake
We suck on a straw and we bake the cake"
– Bluebird & Skoko, "Suck on a Straw"

At the age of 35, when I became pregnant, I didn't have the slightest idea of what the placenta was, how it looked like, what was its functions, how it worked. Did the word include the amniotic sac and the waters? In Croatian, the word for placenta is *posteljica*, "little bed", which gives space for myriad visual interpretations, none of them resembling the actual physical form of the organ itself. All of a sudden, the placenta popped into my life claiming its slice of attention. There wasn't only the baby, there was her placenta too. I was reading all the books I could get to fill the void. I stumbled upon Lotus Birth.

I found the idea of leaving the cord intact and the placenta attached to the baby until it detached spontaneously very fascinating. I immediately felt it was the right thing to do. The list of potential benefits for the newborn was long and convincing. I managed to talk Roberto, my baby's father, into Lotus Birth. Yet, I had no idea how we would take care both of the baby and her placenta once they stayed with us. But, it was an option a baby has only once in her life, and I surely wanted to offer my Koko this chance, whether its benefits were approved scientific truth or just old wives' tales. It was like making one of those elaborate cakes that needed carefully selected ingredients, a delicate hand, and patient non-invasive monitoring while baking, with a final cold sweat while the cake is taken out from the oven. The cake then "needs to rest" – one can't simply and brutally cut it straight away, while all the molecules are still swarming wildly. No, all the patience of this world is needed to make it slowly calm down to its final exquisite shape and taste. Waiting makes it delicious.

Roberto and I decided to give birth to our daughter in Bali, where we lived part of the year. We happen to find out there was an American midwife who was practicing natural birth in Bali. A friend gave us her number so we went to visit Ibu Robin Lim at Bumi Sehat birth clinic near Ubud. When we first spoke to her she told us she was supporting Lotus Birth without knowing we wanted it. Everything she was saying was matching our birth plan. We liked her straight away. Robin was the person I was looking for, I felt like I was in good hands. Now, I could relax. I couldn't imagine explaining to any hospital staff what Lotus Birth was. When we came to Bumi Sehat in labor, we brought a prime quality salt rock to be used for the conservation of our placenta. After my waterbirth, as soon as the placenta came out, Ibu Robin put it in a steel bowl and covered it with fresh flowers she collected on the way to the clinic. It was Bumi Sehat way to give it a loving welcome. Koko was born in the evening. When Robin came back the next morning, she carefully washed the placenta with running water, put it on clean gauze in a basket, and then covered it with salt. It was round and rather heavy, about half a kilo. Disk-shaped, meaty, with widespread vessels like the roots of a tree, it was an uncommon vision. It did resemble a big pancake though, like suggested by its Latin name. It didn't smell bad. However, it made me shredder at the touch – it was so alive. Koko and her placenta were emitting a peculiar fragrance. Ibu Robin likes this scent; she said we should indulge in it too until it lasts - only few days.

Koko's umbilical cord was white, soft and chubby at first. It was protruding from the navel like a cable from an electric guitar. Looking at the little belly of my daughter, I had the impression to stare at some character of Moebius comic books, it was mystic and fantastic. Her red, round and plump navel was embracing the cord like a wedding ring. In two days, the cord drained. It happened suddenly; it collapsed and turned brown in a few hours. Now, there was a less flexible "telephone wire" sticking out of the navel. It became more complicated taking care of the baby and her components. However, the feeling of fragility was only apparent. The navel and the cord were holding tightly to each other while their relationship was obviously drying out. Occasional sudden movements would scare us, but our baby wouldn't even

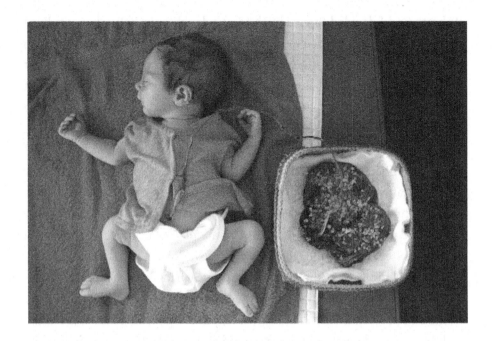

blink. We even managed to put Koko in her sling that I wrapped around me carrying her like a pea, her placenta lying to the side in the basket. When I sat in the car, the cord was extending from the sling to the basket placed on my knees. It survived one hour drive on a bumpy road in a clapped out van. At home, I carefully unwrapped Koko and laid her on the mattress. I was sleeping next to her during night and watching over her by day. In the meanwhile, I was breastfeeding her supinely and changing her diapers often. By the end, the navel was holding on the cord with two tiny slimy threads. We had to pay extra attention on them when we were changing her. Still, those fairy threads were keeping the connection tightly. In the afternoon of the third day, a couple of friends came to visit us. They entered the room at the very same moment when Koko had a big urge. I was about to change her, I glimpsed away in their direction, and then turned back to Koko. I realized her cord was detached. Hurray! Congratulations, Koko, you officially entered your new life. The navel was fine and clean. I landed few drops of my breast milk from time to time, until it was completely closed and dry. The shape of her belly button kept changing for a month or so. After it dried, for some time it looked like Buddha's eye. We were wondering how it would be at the end. We asked Robin, she said it would be like ours. We realized the shape of the navel doesn't change if the cord is cut or not. Even if the cord is cut at birth, there is still a little scrap of it left hanging for a week or more, until it spontaneously drops. Koko now has our concave wheel shaped navel.

When the cord detached, we were left with a shrivelled placenta that we still kept in salt. I put it outside to sun dry. After three days, I carefully tore out the dry cord and put it in a special red bag I crocheted myself when I was waiting. The weather wasn't so propitious for sun drying, the air being far too wet. It was raining season after all. At the end, I oven-dried the remaining placenta until it became a crispy biscuit. It shrunk to one third of its original shape. I took a traditional Indonesian stone mortar and pestle, where they usually crush curry spices. I reduced the placenta biscuit in little chunks, and then grind it into fine powder. I could have used a blender, it would be much easier, but I read it would transfer the sharp and speedy blender spirit into the placenta powder. My placenta cookbook said the way it was handled was very important, since the procedure influences the result, as every cook knows. It was like making a magic potion. The placenta powder is supposed to keep its original beneficial properties for three years if properly kept in the fridge. I used it dissolved in a little water during 40 days of port-partum rest. My placenta tasted exceptionally salty. Its original flavor was altered by the preserving process, but it still tasted somehow organic. There was the option to eat it raw, soon after birth. However, Koko and her placenta were one thing for three days, so I couldn't really give it a bite without feeling like a cannibal. The idea of having an organic medicine made from my own body was thrilling. Koko would continue to benefit from precious nutrients of our placenta through breastfeeding.

Lotus Birth – A Ritual for Our Times

By Sarah J. Buckley

Lotus Birth is the practice of leaving the umbilical cord uncut, so that the baby remains attached to his/her placenta until the cord naturally separates at the umbilicus- exactly as a cut cord does- at 3 to 10 days after birth. This prolonged contact can be seen as a time of transition, allowing the baby to slowly and gently let go of his/her attachment to the mother's body.

Although we have no written records of cultures, which leave the cord uncut, many traditional peoples hold the placenta in high esteem. For example, Maori people from New Zealand bury the placenta ritually on the ancestral marae, and the Hmong, a hill tribe from South East Asia, believe that the placenta must be retrieved after death to ensure physical integrity in the next life: a Hmong baby's placenta is buried inside the house of its birth.

Lotus Birth is a new ritual for us, having only been described in chimpanzees before 1974, when Clair Lotus Day, pregnant and living in California, began to question the routine cutting of the cord. Her searching led her to an obstetrician who was sympathetic to her wishes, and her son Trimurti was born in hospital and taken home with his cord uncut. Lotus Birth was named by, and seeded through Clair to Jeannine Parvati Baker in the US and Shivam Rachana in Australia, who have both been strong advocates for this gentle practice.

Since 1974, many babies have been born this way, including babies born at home and in hospital, on land and in water, and even by caesarean section. Lotus Birth is a beautiful and logical extension of natural childbirth, and invites us to reclaim the so-called third stage of birth, and to honour the placenta, our baby's first source of nourishment.

I am a New Zealand GP (family MD in America), and have 4 children born at home in my adopted country, Australia. I have experienced Lotus Birth with my second and subsequent children, after being drawn to it during my second pregnancy through contact with Shivam Rachana at the Centre for Human

Transformation in Yarra Glen, near Melbourne. Lotus Birth made sense to me at the time, as I remembered my time training in GP obstetrics, and the strange and uncomfortable feeling of cutting through the gristly, fleshy cord that connects baby to placenta and mother. The feeling for me was like cutting through a boneless toe, and it felt good to avoid this cutting with my coming baby.

Through the CHT I spoke with women who had chosen this for their babies, and experienced a beautiful post-natal time. Some women also described their Lotus-Birth child's self-possession and completeness. Others described it as a challenge, practically and emotionally. Nicholas, my partner, was concerned that it might interfere with the magic of those early days, but was happy to go along with my wishes.

Zoe, our second child, was born at home on the 10th of September 1993. Her placenta was, unusually, an oval shape, which was perfect for the red velvet placenta bag that I had sewn. Soon after the birth, we wrapped her placenta in a cloth nappy, then in the placenta bag, and bundled it up with her in a shawl that enveloped both of them. Every 24 hours, we attended to the placenta by patting it dry, coating it liberally with salt, and dropping a little lavender oil onto it. Emma, who was 2, was keen to be involved in the care of her sister's placenta.

As the days passed, Zoe's cord dried from the umbilical end, and became thin and brittle. It developed a convenient 90-degree kink where it threaded through her clothes, and so did not rub or irritate her. The placenta, too, dried and shrivelled due to our salt treatment, and developed a slightly meaty smell, which interested our cat!

Zoe's cord separated on the 6th day, without any fuss; other babies have cried inconsolably or held their cord tightly before separation. We planted her placenta under a mandarin tree on her first birthday, which our dear friend and neighbour Annie later dug up and put in a pot when we moved interstate. She told us later that the mandarins from the tree were the sweetest she had ever tasted.

Our third child, Jacob Patrick, was born on the 25th September 1995, at home into water. Jacob and I stayed in the water for some time after the birth, so we floated his placenta in a plastic ice-cream carton (with the lid on, and a corner cut out for the cord) while I nursed him. This time, we put his placenta in a sieve to drain for the first day. I neither dressed nor carried Jacob at this time, but stayed in a still space with him, while Nicholas cared for Emma, 4, and Zoe, 2. His cord separated in just under 4 days, and I felt that he drank deeply of the stillness of that time.

His short "breaking forth" time was perfect because my parents arrived from New Zealand the following day to help with our household. He later chose a Jacaranda tree under which to bury his placenta at our new home in Queensland.

My fourth baby, Maia Rose, was born in Brisbane, where Lotus Birth is still very new, on 26 July 2000. We had a beautiful 'Do It Yourself' birth at home, and my intuition told me that her breaking forth time would be short. I decided not to treat her placenta at all, but kept it in a sieve over a bowl in the daytime, and in the placenta bag at night. The cord separated in just under 3 days and, although it was a cool time of year, it did become friable and rather smelly (salt treatment would have prevented this). Maia's placenta is still in our freezer, awaiting the right time for burial, and I broke off a piece of her dried cord to give to her when she is older.

My older children have blessed me with stories of their lives before birth, and have been unanimously in favour of not cutting the cord- especially Emma, who remembered the unpleasant feeling of having her cord cut, which she describes as being "painful in my heart". Zoe, at five years of age, described being attached to a 'love-heart thing' in my womb and told me, "When I was born, the cord went off the love-heart thing and onto there (the placenta) and then I came out." Perhaps she experienced her placenta in utero as the source of nourishment and love.

Lotus Birth has been, for us, an exquisite ritual, which has enhanced the magic of the early postnatal days. I notice an integrity and self-possession with my lotus-born children, and I believe that lovingness, cohesion, attunement to nature, trust, and respect for the natural order have all been imprinted on our family by our honouring of the placenta, the Tree of Life, through Lotus Birth.

Lotus Birth: A Mother's Perspective

By Rebecca Bashara

After seeing Inti enter the world bruised, blue and misshapen from squeezing through a passage so tight, my heart had no question about letting him keep his placenta until he was ready to part from it. It felt right to refrain from performing unnecessary procedures on his little body. He had enough work to do, getting used to his body. Scott and I felt that if there was a possibility that his attached cord and placenta could make him feel whole, then we must honor that.

My only preparation for the ritual of leaving our newborn son's cord intact was to read a few essays written by Jeannine Parvati Baker about Lotus Birth. Jeannine wrote from a spiritual perspective; her words conveyed a connectedness and peacefulness in her own babies, who were left intact. But I wasn't prepared for the practical side of it: How do you dress your "connected" baby? How do I nurse and swaddle my boy while he's still connected to his placenta?

We started out by washing the blood from the placenta, then generously applied ground rosemary, even putting the fragrant herb in all the folds. We wrapped the placenta in a disposable diaper and placed it in a basket, just beside us. We were always careful not to move too quickly or pull the cord, which was still a part of our baby. The next day Scott came up with lovingly wrapping the placenta in a cloth diaper and pinning it securely closed. Each day we would unwrap it and change the diaper. In doing this we experienced a silent awe – the miracle of life. We felt the importance of the placenta to our son's health and well-being: he was still being protected and taken care of by his soul brother.

Surreal, our six-year-old daughter, would gather close to us to watch the diapering of her little brother's placenta. She loved to help, and we gave her the important task of lifting the placenta when we were moving Inti from one place to another. She felt so important and so connected. She seemed to understand deeply the reason for leaving her brother's placenta attached. She asked questions about her own placenta. She dreamed of visiting "her" at the tree "she" was planted under. She slipped into the greater mythology of where babies come from. She told me the story of how she chose me to be her mother and of how she was once an angel with beautiful wings. She understood where Inti was before he entered this world. It gave Surreal a connection to her brother, through her own vast subconscious placenta memories, a connection that would last forever.

Surreal would not leave the house while Inti's placenta was still attached. Not even for a tempting play with her friend next door. She didn't want to miss anything and was happy to play quietly while Inti and I slept and recovered from our tumultuous birth. Perhaps in these quiet play times with her dolls, she was rebirthing herself. Maybe she was weaving magical spells to protect her brother. Maybe she was dreaming of her own soul's placenta.

We found that swaddling was the best way to care for the connected cord, so Inti didn't wear clothes for the three days and nights he was still connected. While the placenta wore a diaper, Inti did not, as we did not want anything to rub against the site where his cord was attached. The cord had dried out within the first twelve hours. It began to curl and shape itself into a dance frozen in time. The brittleness of the cord worried me, rubbing up against the baby's fresh skin. So we found ways to swaddle him so that the cord was directed away from his belly. Our only criticism of the Lotus Birth was that we couldn't easily swoop him up and cuddle him against our naked skin without worrying about the cord being pulled. It was three days of total mindfulness.

What did Inti think of being connected? Or how did he feel? Only he knows, but I could say that he was calm and peaceful in the transition into his earthly body. As his cord dried up and the placenta slept in the land between, Inti slept; he dreamt; he grew.

Rebecca Bashara is the mother of two children. She and her husband, Scott, design, sculpt and make jewelry from river stones and silver. She lives in Washington State.

Lotus Birth in Denpasar, Bali

It was full moon when I was called to catch the granddaughter of my dear friend Frederika. Her daughter Ratna had planned to go to the hospital, as her Acehnese, Muslim husband, Hajis, was very conservative, and she did not want to push him out of his comfort zone by planning a home birth.

However, baby Jazmeen had something else in mind. Ratna began early labor as she and Hajis walked on the beach, and only then did she confess that she was not fond of the doctor and hospital they had chosen. They spent the day going from hospital to hospital, looking for a place that felt right. Soon Hajis became sensitive to the negative environment of each place. Ratna could not decide on a birth location, as each time she approached the doors of a hospital, she began to vomit violently and feel increasingly afraid for her baby. Labor progressed and Ratna finally called her mom in tears to confess their problem: now neither parent was convinced that the hospital was a safe place for their baby's birth.

Ratna was shy to call me. She knew that she could have seen me during the pregnancy but had not, as she did not want to build up hopes for homebirth if it was not to be. I was in the middle of 16 year-old Putu's labor, her baby crowning when Frederika, the grandmother-to-be, called. My assistant answered and as it was urgent held the phone to my ear. Ratna was now in active labor at home. After Putu delivered her baby safely, I left her with the Bumi Sehat staff and headed out to Denpasar to evaluate Ratna. Ratna was laboring hard with her wonderful, supportive husband by her side. Less than two hours after I arrived, in the tub with warm water and sprinkled with flowers that had been picked by her father, Ratna gently pushed her baby girl into the world. Baby Jazmeen was greeted by the sweet sound of Adzan, the Islamic call to prayer sung by her father and grandfather.

Hours later, when the subject of the cord and placenta came up, Jazmeen shrieked when her father mentioned cutting the cord. Ratna could not bear to close her heart and asked me if cutting the cord was necessary. I told them they could do Lotus Birth and leave Jazmeen's umbilical cord intact until it fell off naturally. Jazmeen's grandfather loved the idea of ground nutmeg, *pala*, as it is called in Indonesia, being used to dry the placenta.

As the next three days passed, I saw the family bond closer together. They loved their decision to have a Lotus Birth. I left it open for them to change their minds at any time, but they discovered that their baby girl would cry if they even casually suggested cutting her cord. They planted a Jasmine vine over the burial site of the placenta, and that spot never experienced violence.

Ratna and Hajis have had three daughters and are expecting a forth baby. All of their children have been Lotus born. Alhamdulillah!

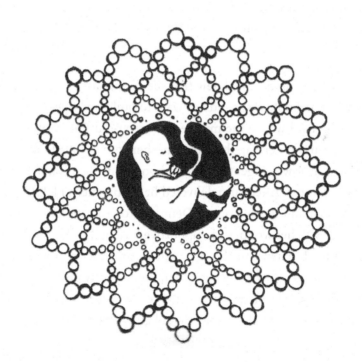

The Internal Grandmother

By Sara Wickham

Amongst the Indian tribes of North America there's a belief that the soul lives in the birth organs; when the cord and the afterbirth have dried up and dropped away they're tenderly gathered up by the mother and arranged in a sacred fabric that she had woven during the pregnancy. This bundle is then buried secretly, and retrieved whenever the tribe moves. This bundle is presented to the grown person when they appear to have children who will survive into adulthood. The mother lays the bundle into the arms of the person with this statement:

> *"Today you are a man, or woman, and I return this to you, for you to look after. I have protected your soul all of your life; now it's up to you."*

It is only in the last few generations of humankind that the placenta has been so carelessly discarded, disregarded, sold on to cosmetic companies or happily left behind, an unpleasant reminder for some of what is perceived as the 'messiness' of birth.

For our great-grandmothers, the placenta would have held a different meaning. Some cultures, as above, regard the placenta as a sacred organ and use this to celebrate spiritual rituals associated with birth and the baby's life. Ancient midwives may have used the hormonal and nutritional strength of the placenta to strengthen the mother after a difficult birth, or to prevent post-partum bleeding or depression.

As in many other birth practices, we are beginning to see a reclamation of ancient traditions and attitudes in the way women and midwives are viewing the placenta, and in the way this organ is being brought into the rite of passage that is birth. Whether women are choosing to bury, eat or retain their placenta, or in some cases to leave this attached to their babies until it falls off naturally, there is a noticeable increase in the way we are becoming more conscious of this incredible organ.

The placenta has been variously described as "the internal grandmother", "the baby's cake" and "the baby's home". It is interesting that many of the different cultures that have ways of celebrating the placenta justify this in relation to their spiritual beliefs. In Thailand the placenta is buried, a ritual that holds deep spiritual meaning for parents. A couple of years ago, I met a Hungarian obstetrician who explained that some of the people she worked with believed that cutting the baby's cord less than six or seven inches from the body was an insult to the baby's aura. She explained that the cord should not be cut less than this distance, because the baby's aura might be harmed as a result.

In other cultures, Lotus Birth is practiced. In this ritual, the umbilical cord is left uncut and the baby and placenta remain as one for several days, until the entire cord and placenta naturally separate from the baby, a few days after birth. Many believe that this allows a more gentle transition for the baby, and enables the child to have an element of choice in when s/he leaves her 'tree of life' and becomes truly independent in the world.

So is Lotus Birth natural? Would our ancestors really have practiced this? One group of midwives I know have historically chosen to cut the cord relatively soon after birth, on the basis that this is what some primates are seen to do.* Would our grandmothers really have left the placenta attached in this way? Is this an ancient ritual, or a relatively new one?

Unfortunately, we cannot say for sure. But, as Michel Odent, author of *The Scientification of Love*, points out in his introduction to "Lotus Birth", we need to re-learn what birth can be like when it is not disturbed, using non-interventive reference points such as Lotus Birth in order to do so.

Often, the midwife will assist the mother in 'preparing' the placenta after the baby and placenta are born. Although there are a number of ways of doing this, the method with which I am familiar involves spreading out a clean towel or nappy, filling this with a mixture of salt and dried herbs (specific herbs may be chosen for their spiritual or medicinal associations) and placing the placenta

---

* See the section *Primates and Placentas* on page 129.

on top of this. More salt and herbs are gently packed on top of the placenta, and the towel is then carefully secured, so that it can be carried around and/or placed next to the resting baby.

One of the most interesting features of Lotus Birth for me is the marked difference which having the placenta attached makes to the degree to which the baby can be passed around to relatives and friends. Although women who choose rituals such as Lotus Birth may also be more likely to practice some degree of postnatal seclusion (or 'babymooning'), there may be an advantage here for the women who are not secluded, yet still end up spending more time with their baby because of the increased difficulty involved in passing a baby around who is still attached to her placenta.

Considering Lotus Birth

By Christina Wadsworth

First published in *The Birthkit* – Vol. 31, Autumn 2001 (a publication of Midwifery Today)

"You mean we don't have to cut it?"

My husband sounded both pleased and surprised. I was pregnant with our third child and we were discussing – not perineums, not foreskins – but umbilical cords.

"Apparently not," I said.

"What happens to it?"

"Supposedly it eventually just dries up and falls off by itself."

"Hunh. Well sure. Let's just not then."

Always an early adapter, my husband had no problem making the leap from homebirth to louts birth. In fact, we both liked the idea of not cutting the umbilical cord at all but letting it fall away in its own time. Every major parenting decision we had made so far – birth at home, not to circumcise, not to vaccinate, home schooling – had both reflected and reinforced our faith in natural processes. Lotus Birth seemed a natural extension of our evolving parenting style. As the primary caregiver and the person with the most questions, however, I still had a bit of research in front of me.

It's amazing how complicated we can make it not to intervene. I had so many questions. I wondered how inconvenient it would be to carry both baby and placenta around. I wondered how badly the placenta would smell as it aged. I wondered what visitors would say. I wondered how long it would take to fall off. I wondered if we would change our minds, or if we could. And although I seldom admitted it, I wondered what the baby's belly button would look like.

The only person I had heard talk about not cutting the cord was a midwife who spike of the baby and placenta as sharing one aura. Although there were no nerves involved, she maintained that the baby experienced the cutting of the cord as something like severing a body part. She was so vehement I was hardly able to get past her personal charge on the subject and listen to what she had to say. And since I had never seen an aura, I felt I had no way of evaluating her claims. However, if it weren't for her we might never have heard of Lotus Birth, and she did tell us that covering the placenta with ground, dried rosemary could forestall any odor problems.

I was able to meet with one of the midwife's clients who had had a Lotus Birth, and the client was very enthusiastic about it. She told me that she felt her youngest child was more calm and at ease in the world as a result of having had a Lotus Birth. She also assured me that it was really very easy to deal with the placenta while waiting for the cord to dry up and drop off. I was reassured but didn't quite work up the courage to ask her what her kid's belly button looked like.

The only written material I was able to find was in Jeannine Parvati Baker's book *Prenatal Yoga and Natural Birth*. It had taken her son's cord about four days to drop off, and that didn't seen too long to endure. Also, I liked what Baker said about letting the placenta fall off in its own time, setting the stage for letting the psyche develop and move on at its own pace. That clinched it for me. Even if it meant carting around something akin to a large piece of liver for a time, we would have a Lotus Birth. I would just have to trust that the baby's belly button would turn out all right.

It seemed like such a big deal going into it, but in reality it was so simple. With midwives standing by, I birthed our son into my hands just one or two contractions after the bag of waters broke. We lingered in the birthing tub until I felt like standing, at which point I birthed the placenta into a small plastic basin. While my husband and I focused on the baby, my mother rinsed the excess blood off the placenta and covered it in ground rosemary. Then she placed it in an old bamboo steamer on top of a plate. When visitors came to see the baby it was very easy just to pop the lid over the placenta.

As the baby and I spent most of the early days in bed, the only tricky part was maneuvering to nurse the baby with his attachment always there. I joked with my stepsister that it was a lot like trying to maneuver to make love when you're nine months pregnant. But I felt the benefits of not having an open wound (a cord stump), and thus no concerns about infection, were fair compensation for this temporary inconvenience. I found myself contemplating the potential benefits of Lotus Birth to babies born in settings where sterile instruments are not so easy to come by.

My stepsister called his placenta "his friend from another planet." And as it dried, a shrinking disk all covered in green powder, it did look rather alien. But our baby seemed content, making the transition gradually from inside to outside the womb.

My mother turned the placenta several times a day, filling and refilling the cracks on the maternal side and the insides of the membranes with ground rosemary. In all, she used nearly four cups of the herb. By day three after the birth the cord had gotten hard and wiry, and although my baby remained physically connected to the placenta, I felt his attachment to the placenta had gone.

I am one of those impatient people who just have to pick at a scab, so the next few days of waiting were hard for me. But I tried to take it as a lesson in parenting and renewed my commitment to letting my baby decide when to move on.

Once around day four, he held the wiry cord in his had for two minutes. His arm was straight up, his hand in a fist. "This could be it," I thought. I held my breath, waiting, until he put his hand down and released his cord. Ha – fooled ya Mom.

By day six the cord was like a loose tooth, hanging by one small, tenuous connection. The baby was kicking and fuming during a diaper change. His foot caught on the cord and "pop" it was off. It didn't seem completely dry yet, so I put golden seal* at his naval and let the winter sun shine through the window and onto his belly.

_____

* Yunan Bai Yao available at Chinese Pharmacies is a nice dry herb, which also works very well to dry up that slightly weepy belly button, weather or not the baby has a Lotus Birth. Just open the capsule and sprinkle some on. – R. L.

For the next few moments my attention was taken up with diapering and nursing. When the baby was finally settled I had time to take in his new appearance. He looked odd to me without his placenta attached – curiously unencumbered and weightless, like an astronaut without his oxygen tank. In that moment I felt I glimpsed something of what the change must have been like for the baby.

About that time I hear my husband walking by in the hall (also placenta free). "You can see why we don't use placentas out here," I told the baby. "We all move around so much, it just wouldn't be convenient. But while you were inside me it sure was useful, wasn't it?"

He smiled, a huge milked-filled baby grin, and immediately fell fast asleep. Somehow it felt like the birthing was finally complete – our boy had made the transition to our world and was here to stay.

Having a lotus bith really changed my viewpoint. While I was pregnant it had seemed so extreme – people often discuss delaying cord cutting, but how could you not cut it at all? And yet now, when I consider the cord, it seems like the first unnecessary surgery, something akin to an episiotomy or circumcision in its general uselessness. And although I am fortunate to live in a time and place where sanitation and clean surgical instruments are not a problem, I have other concerns. I am concerned about the way our society enforces separateness, even from birth. I wonder what the baby learns at the precognitive biochemical level when the hormonal cocktail that floods the mother-baby system during labor is followed by the surgical separation from the placenta he was joined to for nine months? I feel fortunate that our search for a gentler alternative led us to Lotus Birth.

Oh, and our baby's belly button? It's a very cute "innie."

Christina Wadsworth lives in Fairfield, Iowa, with her husband and three children, Devin (7), Erika (5) and Roan (3). In between parenting duties, she writes and teaches prenatal classes.

Roan's Birth - A Grandmother's Story

By Marie Zenack

This was the first water birth for my daughter, Christina, and her husband, Greg. It was their third baby, and all had been born at home. Devin (4½) and Erika (2½), had both seen birth videos, and Christina practiced the "birthing noises" with the children, explaining that the labor noises meant that she would be working hard.

Devin woke up at about 6:00 a.m. Christina had been laboring since 2:00 a.m. She was sitting on a mattress on the floor, not yet in the tub. When Devin came into the room she told him that she thought the baby would come today. Devin asked, "Where's Dad?" Greg was downstairs getting something for Christina. Devin found him and said, "You know what? Mom says she thinks the new baby will come today!"

The midwives were in the house. One had brought her 12 year-old daughter to help with the other children. Our youngest daughter, Samantha, age 25, was in town to help with the new baby. It was a full house, but Christina preferred to labor alone until the last hour, when Greg went in with her. Even the midwives only went in the room to do brief check-ups.

Devin kept peeking in on his mom through the partially opened door. As the labor progressed he ran down to the kitchen and announced, "Mom's barfing!" "Oh, good!" the midwives said, knowing that labor was moving along quickly. Soon Christina felt that the baby was about to be born and she told Greg to get the kids. We all moved quietly into the birthing room, holding and reassuring the toddlers. I smiled at the midwife's young daughter, who was shyly attending her first birth.

With Christina squatting in the tub, we saw the head come out. Christina felt for a cord around the neck. She said, "I don't feel any cord or anything." The midwives suggested that Christina could push, even without a contraction. However, a good contraction came and with Christina bellowing softly, the baby slipped out into Christina's waiting hands. It was so simple and quick, that the midwives said they felt they had done nothing. Of course they had provided the protected space so that everything could be simple. After the birth of baby Roan Michael, Devin, Erika and their father got into the birth tank to have their photos taken with Christina and Roan. The kids were excited, jumping up and down in the water and saying, "It's the new baby!"

The placenta was born about 15 minutes later, and there was a small amount of bleeding along with it. The kids said, "Yuck! Let's get out of here!" so we dried them up and got them dressed while the midwives cared for Mom and baby, who also got out of the tub.

Because Christina and Greg had chosen a Lotus Birth, the cord was not cut. While the midwives cared for Christina and Roan, I washed the placenta and covered it and the cord with powdered rosemary herb. Caring for the living baby and the dying placenta took place side-by-side. Lifting the placenta, we applied a thick coating of rosemary to both sides, and rested it on my bamboo vegetable steamer. We repeated the rosemary applications at least twice daily. The placenta dried and shrunk more each day, giving off only the pleasant smell of rosemary as it ended its days of caring for my grandson.

On day six, Roan held his dried cord in his hand for about two minutes. We wondered, "Will he do it?" But the cord remained, hanging on like a loose tooth. And, surprisingly, there was no rush. We were all getting used to the idea that there is a time in life for everything. Christina continued to maneuver both placenta and baby for nursings, changings, etc. On day seven, Roan kicked in protest to his diaper change and kicked the cord off in the process. It seemed a time for celebration, as it was both a completion and a beginning.

Christina said that, considering the part that rosemary had played in this whole thing, perhaps she would bury the placenta and plant rosemary on top of it. But the cord we saved to shape into a spiral and make into a dream catcher. Since this little cord brought in the energy that nourished Roan's body, it would now guard and filter the dreams that nourish his Spirit.

The Scientist and the Lotus Birth

Pradheep, a Ph.D in biochemistry, was curious to see how nature would handle the relationship between his son and the placenta when he and his wife Priya decided a Lotus Birth for their first child. He also felt spiritually moved to facilitate a non-violent process for his son to enter the world.

When their son Pranavkrshnan and his placenta were born, we brought forth a bowl of warm water and began the preparation of the placenta. First we washed the excess blood away and then dusted the placenta with ground rosemary, turmeric and salt. Gingerly and respectfully, we wrapped the placenta in a diaper while the baby lay naked and warm against his mother, still attached to his little brother placenta.

Over the course of the magical first week of Pranavkrshnan's life, the cord slowly dried as we changed the placenta's diaper and added herbs daily. There was no unpleasant odor. On day five Pranavkrshnan's grandmother made a discovery: she observed that when her grandson nursed, the placenta would pulse. She pointed this out to Pradheep, who was excited and curious about her discovery. When I visited the family, Pradheep could not wait to demonstrate. I was witness to nothing short of a miraculous revelation: even five days after the birth, though the umbilical cord was dry, seemingly lifeless, the placenta was responsive to the baby being nourished at his mother's breasts. In the words of Pradheep, "I am certain that something here is being communicated. I am not fooled by the dry appearance of the cord. Deep in the center there is life. Something essential is being provided to my baby by his placenta."

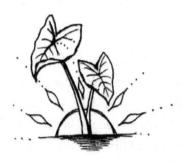

Lotus Birth: A Dad's Perspective

By Mark Ament, A Grateful Papa

When my wife Gabriel and I found out our first baby was on the way, there was no doubt for either of us that we wanted a Louts birth. We had met a lotus born child in New Zealand and she was the most peaceful, confident and happy young child we'd ever met. It seemed obvious to us that her gentle transition into this world contributed to that.

Due to a difficulty with our daughter's umbilical cord, she was born through emergency c-section. Even so, her placenta was attached when she was placed in my arms moments later. I was so happy that her first experiences of the world would be shared with the placenta sister that nourished and protected her during incubation inside and the journey out of the womb.

It was well into the early morning hours when we all made it to our room. Aureya, swaddled in a blanket and perched on my chest, slept peacefully on her side. Her placenta rested nearby, wrapped in a cloth. The next morning when we opened the cloth, I was amazed at the beauty of Aureya's companion. The intricate pattern of veins and vessels seemed to be a combination of brain and heart. I had never seen anything like it, either in nature or from the most creative of imaginations. We carefully set the placenta in a fresh cloth, with ground nutmeg, clove and cinnamon, a bit of salt and few drops of Frankincense essential oil. And then we placed the whole package in a Balinese offering basket.

Over the next days we changed the dressings of the placenta regularly and added more spices - always while Aureya slept or nursed. Aureya seemed to appreciate what was going on by gently smiling often when we handled the placenta. For me it was an honor to perform this little ritual. I felt very happy to do it. In practical terms, having the placenta still attached meant that my wife and I had to move slower and work together when we moved, changed or nursed the baby. It brought all of us closer for the 9 days that the cord remained attached. I believe it gave our family an intimate, gentle and kind start together that surely would have been lost if we had cut Aureya's cord.

On the ninth day, the cord released gently as Aureya was kicking her legs. There was no pain or bleeding at all. My wife and I then honored Aureya and her placenta by burying it under a lime tree, inspired by a similar Balinese custom. The tree has grown nearly 1 meter in the year we've had it and even though it's young, it has been producing fruit regularly.

For me there is simply no alternative to Lotus Birth. Aureya, is a happy and balanced baby. She is quick to smile and hardly ever cries. We regularly get comments on how happy, fun and special she is. For me it's clear that the Lotus Birth contributed to this, because she was able to make her transition in her own time, and she was brought into this world securely and gently and peacefully.

Bodhi's Tree

My grandson, Bodhi Padma Edzra Banjo Bernhardt is a home born, lotus baby. We chose to dust his placenta with nutmeg, the precious spice that is an indigenous healing herb in Indonesia. Bodhi's cord released after only 2 ½ days and his beautiful mother cried, "I'm not ready for him to be so separate. I know he is ready, but I am not." My loving son said, "We will keep Bodhi's placenta here in bed with us, until you feel ready, there is no hurry." The placenta lay beside my grandson for the whole day, and when his mother felt it was time, my son buried it under a Bodhi tree seedling in our garden in Bali. After 3 ½ years the Bodhi tree is huge, taller than our three-story house!

When I see a Lotus Birth baby, gingerly holding her cord, I feel the goodness of leaving them intact. The cord and placenta, the baby's companion in the womb, which sustained the mother and child through pregnancy, has shared the baby's magical prenatal world. Babies are soothed by the humming of their placentas during gestation. Why then are we buying into the medical ritual of severing this bond just at the child and mother's most vulnerable, fragile, and tender moment?

For all the above reasons and many more I cannot articulate in words, I have become convinced that Lotus Birth is an important choice. In August 2010, Dr. Kornia, head of Udayana University School of Medicine in Denpasar, Bali, gave a seminar encouraging delayed clamping and cutting of umbilical cords, assuring the audience that it is not a dangerous practice. He also came out in support of Louts Birth as a viable human right to perfectly non-violent birth. I sat in the audience, Dr. Kornia smiling at me, and I heard my heart singing that Bob Dylan song, "... And the times they are a changing."

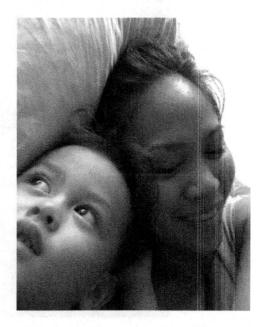

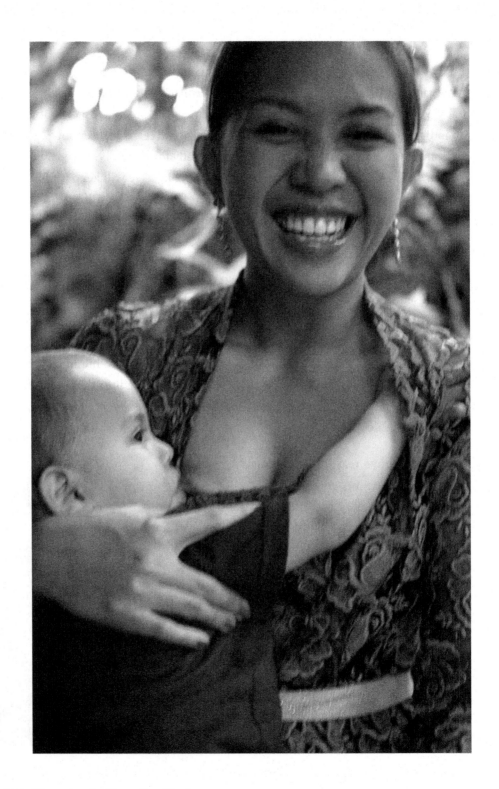

Placentophagy:
Eating the Placenta

"Preparing the placenta for consumption by mothers because of its high protein content is a tradition among Vietnamese and Chinese people."
(National Post, January 12, 1999)

If the idea of eating placenta is revolting to you, ask yourself: How come? A mother's placenta is exactly formulated to give her optimal benefits. No other animal meat will come close to helping her as much as her own placenta. The placenta is so rich in nutrients that it is believed to prevent postpartum depression when ingested. It contains iron and all the minerals that a high-quality meat can offer. Women who have eaten placenta postpartum, either raw to help control/stop hemorrhage, or cooked as a postpartum meal, report feeling brighter and more alert. It is the only meat we can get by giving life, instead of the violence of killing. Why then, is eating placenta considered so disgusting by so many? Eating placenta is not for everyone.

Doctors of traditional Chinese medicine often advise nursing mothers to boil their baby's placenta and drink the broth to improve their milk quality and supply. Human placenta is also used in the preparation of the Chinese medicine Zi He Che.

"The sale and consumption of placenta is common in China, though frowned upon by the authorities. Only those with good connections to the medical world can obtain placenta, which cost between 2.50 and 3.00 pounds Sterling each. According to traditional Chinese medicine, it is regarded as particularly beneficial for a nursing mother to eat her own placenta because it improves her milk. It is usually drunk in the form of a soup." [1]

Eating the placenta as a postpartum tonic is also a tradition in some parts of Vietnam.

Placentophagia is not such an unusual behavior for most mammalian mothers in the perinatal period. Nevertheless, many women of modern cultures do not eat their placentas, as they have a learned response to it: revolting, even associated with cannibalism. How can it be cannibalism, when it is the only meat we can get from birth, rather than meat obtained by killing a sentient being? Animals of all the mammalian groups: carnivores, herbivores and omnivores, those that seek the company of others from their group when they give birth, those who give birth in solitude, those who live in trees or on the ground, most all will ingest the placentas of their newborn young. Animals are not aware of the biochemical benefits, yet instinctually they find the placenta extremely palatable immediately after giving birth. Since there are scientifically documented benefits to eating the placenta, it makes sense that, over time, mammals that eat their placentas thrive in the process of natural selection; they enjoy an adaptive biological advantage.

"Why most mammalian mothers eat the afterbirth during delivery is still a mystery...in fact, a double mystery. We are not sure either of the immediate causes, although presumably the material becomes very attractive in smell and taste at that time; nor are we sure of the consequences of the behavior. The consequences, of course, if beneficial, must have affected evolution in such a way as to provide for the internal substrate that accounts for the immediate causes, and thereby must be considered the ultimate cause of the behavior. For instance, because of an adaptive advantage conferred on mothers that ate placenta during

delivery, or on their offspring, selection pressure would eventually increase the frequency of parturitional placenta-eaters in the population. Thus, the beneficial consequences of ingesting the afterbirth will have produced populations of animals that find placenta extremely palatable. To the individual, the immediate causes of eating the afterbirth during the first delivery must necessarily be that it looks good, tastes good, smells good, or feels good. The animal itself is certainly unaware of adaptive consequences of the act." [2]

It is interesting that animals who eat their placentas do not eat their helpless young, although the placenta smells, tastes and is genetically identical to the newborn mammal.

"The Navaho treated the placenta as sacred, but also as poisonous; the Kol believed that if the placenta were eaten by the mother, she would die. The Shilliuk, apparently practicing symbolic ingestion of the afterbirth, buried the placenta at the roots of a fruit tree, then during the next season ritualistically ate the fruit or drank tea brewed from the fruit. It remains possible that placentophagia is practiced in some cultures, or may have been before the era of modern anthropological records..." [3]

For many years I kept Nubian milk goats. These gentle creatures were absolutely vegetarian, except for the females, who ate meat once a year after giving birth. After kidding (goat giving birth), the mother goats would deliver the placenta and immediately eat it raw. It was these goats, free of the cultural hang-ups and judgments that taught me that eating placenta was a natural craving for mammals. By ingesting the meat of the placenta, the new mother is able to replace the minerals from the blood loss of birth. The vitamins and protein ease the strain of the long months of pregnancy on the mother's body and balance her plummeting hormone levels. This organ that supports the living baby in the mother's womb, if eaten, further supports the offspring by insuring an adequate and flowing milk supply.

Pharmaceutical medicines are a miracle when needed and available, but they do have side effects. A woman who is given oxytocin drugs, methergine (both by injection) or misoprosol to control hemorrhage will experience an imbalance in her body. Hormones are powerful; the postpartum woman, in the best of circumstances, is coping with a lot of adjustments and re-balancing in the first precious hours and days after having a baby. Injecting drugs may be necessary to save the mother's life, but how much better is it to use the new mother's own natural resource to protect and heal her?

According to German midwife, Cornelia Enning, author of the book *Placenta the Gift of Life*, ingesting placenta for medicinal purposes postpartum has been practiced for generations throughout the world. This knowledge has been passed down for generations, but in modern times it is frowned upon. The use of pharmaceutically prepared, injectable oxytocic drugs to control hemorrhage after childbirth has caused the use of ingesting placenta as an essential medicine in the preservation of maternal life to be deemed unnecessary.

For the woman who has suffered high blood pressure, edema (swelling of the legs, feet, and/or hands) and has had protein in her urine during pregnancy, ingesting some of her own placenta heals and soothes her kidneys and helps resolve these symptoms more quickly. It can also be used as a natural medicine for pain that occurs shortly after delivery:

> *"The most general benefit of placentophagy, according to recent research, is that placenta and amniotic fluid contain a molecule (POEF, Placental Opioid-Enhancing Factor) that modifies the activity of endogenous opioids in such a way that produces an enhancement of the natural reduction in pain that occurs shortly after and during delivery."* [4]

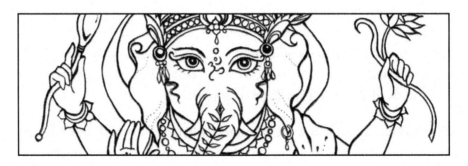

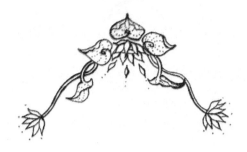

Eating the placenta also helps mothers breastfeed, and, according to traditional Chinese medicine, it can be used to treat insufficient lactation.[5] Mothers who have had Toxemia or preeclampsia during pregnancy may find their milk slow to come in. This can take the joy out of lactation; the swelling from toxemia can take many weeks to resolve. By eating her placenta this woman's symptoms will be more quickly alleviated and her milk more likely to flow normally by the third day postpartum.

> "The placenta is a "privileged graft": the fetal placenta (and indeed, the fetus), is immunoincompatible with the mother by virtue of antigens inherited from the father, yet the fetal placenta and fetus are obviously not rejected under normal circumstances. The mother's immunological system is, however, permanently altered by gestation, due to the migration of fetal erythrocytes across the placenta or during delivery. In certain cases, the first pregnancy may immunize the mother against fetal antigens present in a subsequent pregnancy. These cases of mother-fetus immunological rejection, such as graft-vs-host disease, or, in humans, erythroblastosis fetalis (Rh-incompatibility), can result either in death of the fetus or neonate, or in severe physical and mental impairment. The disorders are brought about by the formation of antibodies to the fetal antigens in the antigen-deficient mother. That placenta contains factors which, if ingested during delivery, would prevent the mother from forming the antibodies, becomes an intriguing candidate for the elusive adaptive advantage. We may not have to look far for the active substances; even estrogen and progesterone, found in abundance in the placenta, suppress the immunological processes involved in tissue rejection."
>
> – Mark B. Kristal, from *Placentophagia: A Biobehavioral Enigma*

Benefits of eating the placenta for all mammals – including humans!

- Increased effectiveness of mother-infant bonding

- Reduction of postpartum hemorrhage

- Protection from ill effects of placental cells that may remain in uterus after birth

- Replenishment of mother's nutrients

- Immunological advantages*

- Documented experiences link ingestion of placenta to a reduction of symptoms associated with postpartum depression

- Supports lactation

- Reduces the mother's pain after childbirth

- Cleans the den to keep predators from smelling the afterbirth and threatening the pups

- Because animal moms lick the baby and the sac while ingesting the placenta, it reduces likelihood newborn will suffocate inside the amniotic sac

Most of the men I have discussed eating placenta with over the years, have expressed disdain. The very thought of eating an organ that issues forth from the vagina of a woman was unthinkable to them. Yet each of them admitted that they enjoyed oral sex with their female lover. Most of them had no qualms about eating organ meats, and indeed they would eat the hearts, livers, even kidneys and brains of cows, pigs, chickens, turkeys and other animals. Perhaps, as men, having never enjoyed the hormonal cocktail of birth and becoming a mother, they therefore could not tolerate the thought of ingesting placenta.

———————

*In addition to the possible milk-born immunological benefits to the suckling neonate, and the possible protection to the mother from becoming immunized against fetal antigens, there is a third route by which placentophagia may be immunologically beneficial. Rather than prevent the mother from becoming immunized, ingestion of placenta may actually effect an immunization -- that of the mother against placental cells remaining in utero after delivery, and which may, if not rejected, eventually pose a threat to the mother's health (e.g., choriocarcinoma).[6]

A 1998 a British television cooking show, *TV Dinner*, featured a family in London preparing and eating the placenta of their newest family member. They fried the placenta with garlic and shallots, pureed it into a pâté, flambéed it, served on focaccia bread. The British Broadcasting Standards Commission received so many complaints from viewers that they finally ruled the program had breeched a taboo that "would have been disagreeable to many."[7] A *Saturday Night Live* skit with comedian Guilda Radner was canceled due to the content: "Placenta Helper," a spoof on the marketing of a product that makes hamburger more tasty. Placenta was considered too sensitive a subject, too revolting to be funny. A *Time Magazine* piece published Friday, 03 July 2009 by Joel Stein, *Afterbirth: It's What's for Dinner*,[8] really had me laughing. In fact, there is now such a variety of reading about placentophagia on the internet that it is an indicator of how minds are opening to the benefits outweighing the taboo. I recently read a satirical article about Tom Cruise' real plans to cook and eat placenta after the birth of his baby: He shares recipes too![9]

Virgin mammals that have not given birth are not attracted to eating placenta, therefore it makes sense that the attraction to eating placenta is a natural side-effect of childbearing and has been selected for, over the millennia.

> *"The striking fact that even those rats that avoid placenta as virgins become enthusiastic placenta eaters during their first delivery suggested to us that endocrine or other physiological changes during pregnancy may shift the attitude toward placenta in much the same way that they facilitate the rapid onset of pup-oriented maternal behaviors (retrieval of young to the nest, pup-licking, crouching over pups) in the immediate-prepartum period."*[10]

I have observed that midwives who have never had a baby are repulsed by the very thought of new mothers eating the placenta, even if ingesting a bit of the placenta may save the mother's life (i.e. in the case of sever postpartum hemorrhage). However, midwives who have given birth are ok, for the most part, with the idea, even with the practice of using placenta as an oral medication and dietary supplement. I did meet one mother/midwife who was extremely opposed to allowing the new mothers to eat any part of their placentas. This midwife was an adoptive mom who never gave birth.

I ate my placentas. I have eight children, five were born from my body, and three were given to me for free, via adoption and marriage. The placentas of the first two children I bore were buried. Déjà, my thirty-four year old daughter can visit her placenta in a beautiful flower garden in Santa Barbara, California. Noël, my son of thirty years, will find his placenta under a peach tree, also in Santa Barbara. When daughter Zhòu was born twenty-five years ago, my midwife, Sunny, offered to cook the placenta for me. She cut away the veins and arteries, which we buried in our garden in Maui, Hawaii. Next, she sautéed the best parts of the placenta with herbs and sweet onion and ground it with breadcrumbs to make the most delicious pâté I have ever tasted. I ate my placenta, spread on toasted bread. At the time I was a vegetarian! Placenta pâté and some fruit were the only foods I wanted in my first few days postpartum. When it was finished, I cried, as if I would starve without this amazing food. My baby's father and my first two children also enjoyed the feast. Even my dear friend, Margo, who struggled with feelings of both revulsion and curiosity, partook of eating my placenta. To this day the bond between us grows strong beyond the boundaries of ordinary friendship.

After my fourth and fifth births, we also cooked and ate the best parts of the placentas. The uneaten remains of my son Zion's placenta rests under a Rainbow Shower tree in upcountry Maui. My youngest son Hanoman's placenta is buried in the family compound where he was born, in Bali.

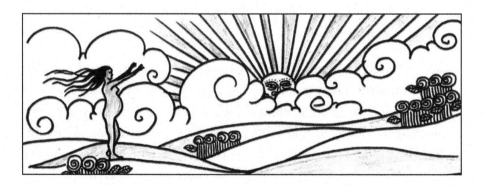

Dani's Testimonial

After my first baby, I had bad postpartum depression, and my doctor put me on anti-depressants. Though it probably saved my life and that of my baby's, taking the medication meant that I had to stop breastfeeding, which I was not keen to do. The additional work of making bottles was awful, and it wore me out getting up at night to go to the kitchen and make bottles, instead of just rolling over in bed and giving baby David my breast.

I also became annoyed with my husband, even though he was working hard to support me through this difficult time. He would do all the getting up for changing and feedings, and he worked extra shifts to pay for all the therapy I needed for my depression. At one point, we almost broke off our marriage. Then, the worst thing I could have imagined happened: I fell pregnant again. I thought it was the end of the world.

When I shared the news with one of my girlfriends, who I affectionately call Hippie, she suggested I meet with a midwife named Sally. Hippie had had a homebirth with Sally and said that her experience changed the way she felt about birth. In desperation, I made the phone call.

Sally was very professional, but also extremely warm. My spirits lifted during our first meeting and continued to improve as my pregnancy progressed. I developed a love and respect for Sally, and that bond I felt with her helped carry me through the remaining months of my pregnancy

At first, I did not tell her about my postpartum depression, because I was afraid she would talk me out of a homebirth, which I was determined to have after hearing Hippie rave about her experience. When I finally did reveal my depression with her, she responded calmly. She suggested we dry, powder and encapsulate my baby's placenta after the birth, and take this as one would take medication.

Well, we did just that. I ate my placenta, which made my friend Hippie laugh. She didn't even try that! I had no symptoms of postpartum depression, unless I forgot to take my placenta pills for two days. What a difference! I am still breastfeeding my toddler. My husband is so happy, he is telling his friends to have their kids at home and eat the placenta!

Maui Midwife Placenta Story

A close friend and midwife from Maui, Jan Francisco, learned during a visit with me in Bali that we used the placenta to control hemorrhage. (In Hawaii, they call the placenta *iewe*.) She was fascinated by this practice and wanted to incorporate it into her midwifery practice in Hawaii. Soon after she returned home, she got the chance. She was helping a homebirth mother birth her second child, this mom had a history of hemorrhage. Though the birth went without complication, the mother hemorrhaged dangerously, postpartum. Jan began by giving her the Chinese patent medicine, Yunnan Bai Yao, and the bleeding stopped. However, after only 20 minutes, the new mother began bleeding again. Jan administered 1cc of pitocin inter-muscularly and the bleeding stopped. Unfortunately, 20 minutes later, the bleeding resumed again. Each time the bleeding returned, Jan administered Chinese herbal medicine or pitocin, as was her normal practice. Each time, the medicine worked for only a short time before the mother's uterus became boggy and profuse bleeding began again.

After four hours, the new mom's blood pressure was dropping, Jan asked the mother if she was willing to eat a piece of her own placenta. The young mother agreed, desperate to end the life-threatening bleeding. "I chose the nicest, loveliest, biggest codelydon and fed it to her, and the mother admitted that it was not bad at all," Jan reported. With this, the bleeding stopped completely and did not resume. The mother later commented that she felt much better than she had after her last birth and that she also felt she would eat placenta after all her future births!

Primates and Placentas

In their scholarly piece *An Observed Birth in a free-living Chimpanzee (Pan troglodytes schweinfurthii) in Gombe National Park, Tanzania,* Jane Goodall and Jamanne Athumani describe the following:

> "On eight occasions mothers were seen when their babies were only one day old or less. Three times the placentas had not been eaten and were carried along with the infants. The female Winkle ate the placenta of her first born – when the nest was examined, after she had left, there was no sign of it. In the four remaining cases the placentas had disappeared and may have been eaten." [11]

This reports that Chimpanzee mothers practice both placentophagia and Lotus Birth!

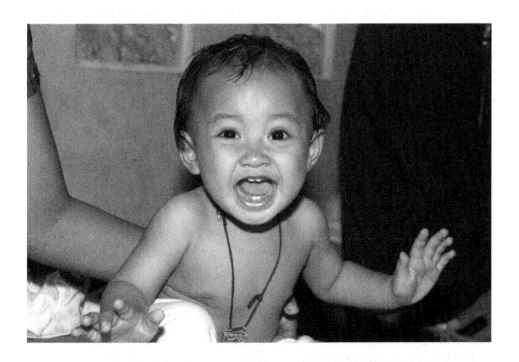

Preparing the Placenta

When preparing placenta for eating or to make medicinal capsules, it is important to rinse the organ well to remove excess blood. I am told by HIV/AIDS experts that once the blood is exposed to air, the virus cannot survive, yet I recommend that women eat only their own placentas, to be safe. If they are disease free, they may wish to share the meal with their family.

Placenta should be no more than 2 to 3 days old when prepared for ingesting. It is best if it is prepared and eaten the very day of the birth. This is not possible with Lotus Birth, but it is still possible to use the placenta by preparing it using the Chinese medicine method. If you cannot cook the placenta on the first day, refrigerate, as you would any fine meat. Remove the tough parts, any calcifications (calcifications will be present only if the baby came a bit late), arteries and the vein, the membranes, as well as the caul. These parts are easily recognizable. Like any fine meat you will wish to cook and eat only the best parts. Make a lovely ritual to bury the remainder of the placenta with respect.

Preparing Placenta the Traditional Chinese Medicinal Way

According to midwife and doctor of Chinese medicine, Raven Lang, the placenta, in traditional Chinese medicine, is considered a powerful sacred medicine, full of life force. To prepare the placenta according to traditional Chinese medicine, wash away the excess blood and place it in a steamer, shiny side down. Steam on low heat for about 15 minutes. Turn and steam 15 more minutes. You will know it is done if no blood comes out when you prick it with a fork. Next slice the placenta into thin, ⅛ inch strips. Place the strips on a cookie sheet and bake in the oven on the lowest possible setting. Several hours later, when the placenta strips are completely dry, like beef jerky, you can grind it with a mortar and pestle or in a food processor or coffee grinder. The powder can then be encapsulated in gel or vegetarian capsules.[12]

Some midwives and mothers prepare the placenta using a food dehydrator rather than an oven. There is some discussion about making medicine capsules with a Lotus Birth placenta that has been salted. Some of the placentas of Lotus Birth families I have helped, which have been salted and in some cases dusted with powdered nutmeg, have also been made into medicine capsules after the cord released, some days following the birth. The mothers ingested these capsules and all three have reported feeling stronger from it. In one case, a mother who had suffered from depressions all her life, and feared postpartum depression, would take two placenta capsules whenever she felt depression coming on. "The placenta helped me, I could feel my mood changing from dark to enthusiastic about life. I'm so happy I have this medicine."

Postpartum and menopausal women find it beneficial to take two or three capsules of their own prepared placenta two or three times a day. Placenta can ease any trauma from a difficult birth, especially if the mother has hemorrhaged. It is especially useful to abating or avoiding postpartum depression.

While preparing the placenta in this way, remember to have reverence, as it is a sacred medicine and indeed a Chakra. The person preparing the placenta should be in good health: of heart, mind and body, as she is transmitting her energy into the placenta. I recommend that any placenta capsules not quickly consumed be stored in the freezer.

Eating Placenta Raw

In case of emergency (i.e. maternal postpartum hemorrhage and/or shock), pull off a nice cotyledon or two from the newly born placenta, leaving it connected to baby by the umbilical cord. Coat this raw bit of placenta with honey and give to mother to drink with water or other room temperature liquid.

Can I still eat my placenta if I choose Lotus Birth?

Yes you can! Many mothers I have helped have taken a small piece of the placenta immediately after birth and eaten it, even if they choose not to sever the umbilical cord. This first bit of placenta food/medicine is more palatable if dipped in honey and/or powdered cinnamon. Both taste good and enhance digestion.

Can I still make my Lotus Birth placenta into medicine for later use?

Salting Lotus Birth placenta not only reduces the odor to nearly nothing, it preserves the placenta so that once the cord releases, it may be used as medicine. This is accomplished by steaming the placenta, slicing it and drying it. Next it is pulverized and put into capsules. It may then be kept in a cool dry place (freezer is best) and used over the course of the postpartum, or even to reduce symptoms of the mother's menopause later in her life. Complete instructions for preserving placenta as in Traditional Chinese medicine is on page 130.

Do something that nobody else has done,

something that will dazzle the world!

– Paramahansa Yogananda 1893 ~ 1952

"I am the Fanua"
by: Fa autu Talapusi
special thanks to Asuka Hirabe

I am the fanua
The placenta buried in my ancestral land after childbirth I am the pute
The umbilical cord buried and my link to my fanua

I am the fanua
The land which holds my history, my life, my death I am the fanua
The land of my people, my ancestors, my descendents

I am the fanua
That which bonds me to the air, the earth, the sea
I am the fanua
That which binds me to the plants, the animals, the fish

I am the fanua
My mother's pain and joy in giving life I am the fanua
Mother earth's pain and joy in giving life

I am the fanua
God's beautiful and unparalleled creation I am the fanua
God's undying and steadfast love

I am the fanua
Wailing in despair at my self-destruction I am the fanua
Dying of a slow suicide

I am the fanua Expecting God's revelation I am the fanua
Believing in God's promise

I am the fanua You are the fanua We are the fanua.

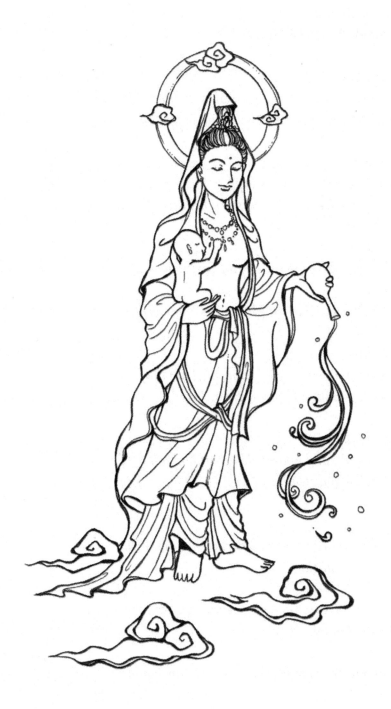

134 *Placenta, the Forgotten Chakra*

Placenta Recipes

Indonesia's most beloved female rock star, Oppie Andaresta was told by many doctors that her baby was so "precious" that she should have a cesarean delivery. Oppie was concerned that surgical birth could jeopardize breastfeeding; Indonesian babies are statistically 300 times more likely to die in their first year of life if they are fed infant formula. Oppie was concerned that the hundreds of thousands of young girls who idolized her, would be influenced away from breastfeeding, if her baby was ever seen with a bottle in his mouth. She decided that a natural vaginal birth was important for her and her baby, as well as, for her fan's future offspring.

To give herself the best chance of having a natural birth with immediate breastfeeding start-up and support, Oppie chose to have her baby with the midwives at Bumi Sehat Bali. She and her husband Kurt arrived quietly, three weeks before her baby's birth.

Oppie sang her baby Earth-side in a pool of water and flowers, surrounded by the midwives she trusted, in a birth clinic that mostly serves the poorest and most underprivileged families. Outside, dozens of well-wishing young fans waited quietly, to see if Oppie would birth naturally and breastfeed.

Kai Bejo was left intact with his umbilical cord and placenta for nine hours, then the cord was burned free. Kurt, the new father, and my husband Wil cooked the best parts of the placenta for Oppie. They flavored it with the vegetables and spices available in my kitchen, and served it in a bowl of red rice. Oppie and Kurt enjoyed every bite.

Kai's umbilical cord was made into a dream catcher. The parts of the placenta not eaten were taken home to Java, to be buried on family land. Kai was exclusively breastfed for six months. Ibu Oppie then combined breastfeeding with healthy foods. She continues to inspire Indonesia's youth as a wonderful, caring, natural, singing Mama.

Placenta Spaghetti Bolognaise

Ingredients:

- **2 tablespoons olive oil**
- **The best parts of 1 fresh placenta** (5-7 oz. or more) cut into small cubes or ground.
- **3 to 4 cloves peeled crushed garlic**
- **1 sweet onion halved and diced**
- **8 oz. fresh sliced mushrooms of your choice** (optional)
- **1-3 teaspoons fresh or dried Italian herbs of your choice:** oregano, thyme, rosemary or bay leaf. If you have a garden, this is the best place to get the herbs.
- **1½ kilo (about 3 lbs.) fresh tomatoes** braised in boiling water to remove peels, then diced (or 8-12 oz. organic tomato sauce of your choice)
- **Healthy Pasta of your choice cooked al dente.**

Preparation:

1. In a large, deep pan, heat oil over medium heat.
2. Add placenta (cubed or ground), garlic, onion, mushroom. Stir while cooking about 5 minutes, until placenta is cooked through and onions are tender.
3. Add tomatoes, lower heat and cover. Simmer for approximately 1 hour (less cooking time if you use a prepared tomato sauce). Add salt to taste.
5. Prepare pasta of your choice.
6. Serve over pasta with a nice side salad.

Placenta Pâté

This recipe is as close as I can come to the delicious pâté that my midwife Sunny Supplee prepared for me after I had my daughter Zhouie at home. Years after Sunny passed away, my husband Wil made a very yummy wonderful pâté from my son Hanoman's placenta. Give it a go!

Ingredients:

- **3 - 4 tablespoons olive oil**
- **1 large shallot**, peeled and coarsely chopped (2 ½ tablespoons). You may substitute with sweet onion
- **The best parts of 1 fresh placenta** (5-7 oz. or more) cut into 1-inch pieces
- **¼ – ½ teaspoon herbes de Provence** (or make your own herb mix, like a pinch each of rosemary, tarragon, basil, oregano, marjoram, etc. We found the garden was the best place to gather the herbs - depending upon the season of your birth.)
- **2 cloves garlic, peeled and crushed**
- **¼ teaspoon salt** (or to taste)
- **¼ teaspoon freshly ground black pepper**
- **1 ½ - 2 teaspoons cognac or sherry**
- **16 pieces of ¼-inch-thick horizontal slices from a small baguette**, toasted, or homemade bread warm from the oven

Preparation:

1. Place olive oil in a skillet, warm on medium to high heat, do not allow oil to smoke.

2. Add the shallots/onion, cook for about 1 to 2 minutes, stirring occasionally.

3. Add the placenta, herbs and garlic, and cook over medium to high heat for 3-4 minutes, stirring occasionally.

4. Add the salt and pepper. It will smell wonderful.

5. Transfer the mixture to a blender, add the Cognac or sherry and blend until smooth/liquefied. This will yield ½ cup. Let cool for at least 1 ½ hours, cover and refrigerate until serving time.

6. Spread the pâté on homemade bread or the toasted baguette slices, and serve. The pâté will keep 3 to 4 days if covered and refrigerated.

Placenta Stroganoff

This is a recipe made famous by our friend Rick Bickford when his wife Danya had her third baby, Chandrika. He garnished his delicious invention with pitted kalamata olives!

Ingredients:

- 2 tablespoons olive oil
- **The best parts of 1 fresh placenta** (5-7 oz. or more) cut into thin strips
- **1 sweet onion halved and diced**
- **½ cup fresh green onion diced**
- **8 oz. fresh sliced mushrooms of your choice**
- **1 red or yellow bell pepper,** core removed and cut into small cubes
- **½ to ¾ cup sour cream**
- **¼ to ½ tsp fresh dill weed finely diced** (may substitute dried dill weed)
- **Pitted whole or sliced kalamata olives** as optional garnish
- **Salt to taste**
- **Healthy whole grain pasta or rice of your choice**

Preparation:

1. In a large skillet heat oil, over medium heat.

2. Add placenta strips, onion, mushroom, red or yellow bell pepper. Stir while cooking about 7 minutes, until placenta is cooked through and onions are tender.

3. Turn off fire and stir in sour cream and dill weed. Salt to taste.

4. Prepare pasta al dente or your choice of rice.

5. Serve stroganoff over prepared pasta or rice, garnished with green onion and olives.

Happy Birthday!

Every year we celebrate our birthdays. It is the completion of our personal journey around the sun, the center of our solar system. Beginning on the day of our birth, we circle this celestial body of light, completing one cycle when once again our date of birth comes around.

On this day of passage into a new solar cycle, we receive a birthday cake. A sweet gift we light with candles and gather around with family and friends. In the light of the candles burning on our birthday cake, we sing out joyfully and share as a community.

Though the tradition of the birthday cake has survived the test of time, the origin and reason for it has been lost to our memories. According to the late Jeannine Parvati, who extensively studied the psychology, history and sociology of birth, the beloved birthday cake was invented by the Druids. It was traditionally round and covered with cherries or red berries and was the symbol to honor our placentas. The wise women who kept the knowledge of the Druids believed that by celebrating the placenta, as each member of our community ate a delicious piece of it symbolically in the form of the cake, we blessed our lives forward, for another year.

Year after year we light candles on our birthday cake, we sing and then we blow out the light. Once I understood that the birthday cake represents our placenta, and that the candles represent the cord, it became disturbing to blow out the candles. Since then, in my family, we put the birthday candles on a small plate on the birthday cake (placenta proxy) sing and leave the candles lit on the plate while we share the cake. In this way we acknowledge long life, by not blowing out the fire, the symbol of life. This feels much more comfortable for this particular mom, who is hyper tuned into placentas and their meaning.

In Latin "placenta" is the word which means a flat round cake
"It may not be pretty to look at, but it's the most beautiful organ
there is. In the Old Testament it was thought to be the External
Soul. In 1559 a man named Realdus Columbus called it
"placenta," after the Latin word for circular cake.
– Williams Obstetrics (18th edition)

Gina's Placenta Poem
by Robin Lim, 1998

To give birth,
choose a starry night
in the Philippine rainy season.
Cut from your new daughter's tree
of life only the choice meat.
Bury the rest with flowers and incense
on your mother's land.
Slice it thin.
Sauté in sesame oil and salty soy,
with one small red onion
and three cloves of garlic - this aroma
Recalls her strength.

Cube and steam one large carrot
and one whole sweet potato, she needs roots here.

Add the roots to the meat
with a pinch of rosemary,
a dash of nutmeg and ground oregano.
One handful of cilantro leaves, so she will wonder.
Two handsfull of leafy greens, because she bled.
Now the juice of five tiny *Kalamansi* lemons.
so she won't fear the sour.
Serve with brown rice
because she's so hungry

More Talk Story

Joe's Placenta

I still remember the day I first met Jan. I was living in Maui at the time. She was pushing her infant son Joseph in a stroller, and Joe was beaming like a burning bush. I got on my knees and kissed him, introduced myself to him and then to his mother. Little did I know that Jan was also a midwife. She would become my dear sister and friend and even receive my next baby, Zion. It would also be Jan who would save me when my life fell apart a few months later.

At the time of my life's meltdown, I found myself a single mother with four children and nowhere to live. When I showed up at Jan's late for dinner with my children, our luggage, a laundry basket, a change of clothing and the manuscript for my first book, they welcomed us with open arms. It was not a big house, but Jan, her husband David and their four children invited us to live with them until I could get back on my feet.

During this time of change for my family, Jan's family was about to move from a rental house and onto the land where they would build their own home. Together we packed all their family belongings and cleaned the house for the next occupants. I found a house of my own, so Jan, David and their four children moved in with me, while they waited for their new house to be built. They spent most of their time living between a small house, a converted school bus parked on my land and outdoors in the garden.

One sunny afternoon I asked Jan, "Whatever did we do with Joe's placenta when we moved?" Since Joe had been born in a rental, Jan had frozen his placenta, so they could bury it on their land. When we moved house together, we had left the frozen placenta for last.

As the question left my lips, Jan froze, "Get the kids in the car," she yelled. Soon we were making the fifteen minute trip from Haiku to Makawao, headed toward Jan's old house. We arrived and nervously knocked on the door. We must have been a sight, two babies and a load of children standing on an all too familiar doorstep. A tall man in his mid-thirties answered the door. We explained that we were the former tenants, and that we had left something precious and important in the freezer. "Well," said the man, "the only thing you left behind was this piece of meat. It looked pretty good, so I thawed it out, and was just about to cook it up for our dinner." Jan gasped and ran toward the kitchen. There on the kitchen counter was Joe's partially defrosted placenta!

We thanked the nice man, explained that this particular piece of meat had special meaning and value. He laughed as he let us out, never knowing that he nearly ate placenta for supper.

Joe's placenta finally found its resting place under a rainbow shower tree, in Haiku, Maui, on their family land. My son Zion was born later that year, and I ate the best parts of his placenta. The remainder was also laid to rest with prayers and songs and flower offerings under the same blooming tree with Joe's placenta.

Mangku Ketut Liyar,
a Love Story and a Small Mistake

I first met Mangku Ketut Liyar – Kak Mangku (literally Grandfather priest) in 1993. This elderly Hindu priest from the small village of Pengosekan was full of spirit and magical knowledge; not yet made famous by the book/film *Eat Pray Love*. He had been, what I like to call, a "Birth Keeper." Before hospitals were accessible in rural Bali, this man was a *Dukun Bayi*, a healer who received babies into the world. He is also a scholar of the *Lontar*, the sacred books of Bali written in *Purwa Aksara* Sanskrit on pages made from the dried leaves of the *lontar* palm; The pages were then bound together with two strings and closed in lengths of bamboo.

After my last birth child and his companion spirit exited my body, our adopted Balinese family brought the baby's offerings to Kak Mangku to be blessed. The family told him nothing of the circumstances of this offering, but when Kak Mangku came out of trance, he told them this, "Oh, you allowed foreigners to have their baby in your traditional home. This child is Balinese, so he was confused to open his eyes and see these strange pale people! The boy must have all the proper Hindu ceremonies. He will be very musical, very tall. Oh, but I'm sorry, he will have very ugly hair!"

My son, Wayan Hanoman is seventeen years old now. He is tall, plays the fiddle like the devil and sings like an angel. Also, he has very red hair, which for the Balinese is considered an ugly demon color!

As I got to know Kak Mangku, he showed me the *Lontar* books, which his family had safe kept for nine generations. Before that, he was not sure where the books came from. Inside he read characters scratched with a knife in an age long past, the letters were wiped with ash, so they could be read. This Balinese writing was in a version of the language so old, that few people remained on earth who could still read it. He showed me the Bali Hindu Dharma instructions for creating ceremonies and rituals to protect children. He showed me the ancient teachings about herbs to aid in childbirth, and where it warned against quickly severing the umbilical cord of a newborn baby.

He showed me how the books could be used to divine who a child had been in a past life, and what this child required in this life to be happy. Over the years I came often to visit Kak Mangku, especially on *kajeng kliwon,* the special day of the Balinese month when healing was more powerful, and on Saraswati Day, when the Goddess of Knowledge was honored and the *Lontar* books were blessed.

I once took my friend Steve to have his daughter Serena blessed on the 12th day of her life. Traditionally the baby is not brought to the priest or priestess for blessing, but offerings are presented instead. The baby must stay at home, and lay-in with the mother, resting and breastfeeding, while the family handles all responsibilities, including the spiritual. Kak Mangku made small talk with Steve and I and even offered his standard, "Do you want your palm read?" line. Then he got down to the ringing of his beautiful bell, and splashing of holy water in a cloud of incense smoke. Finally, he took down the ancient book, my favorite one, which teaches humans how to care for their children. There he read the ancient *Purwa Aksara,* searching the pages for the day and conditions surrounding this baby's birth. He seemed agitated, and took down another book, shaking his head and pouring over the pages. He wrote down some letters in Sanskrit with a leaking ballpoint pen on a scrap of paper torn from a school notebook, and fussed over translating each Sanskrit letter into our modern alphabet.

"Mr. Steve, your baby has two souls," he said. We were surprised, confused and doubtful.

"I checked it here, because I felt it was not possible," he pointed at the other book he had consulted. "This is the first time I have seen a child with two souls incarnate in a female body. Normally, souls who incarnate together like this, in a shared body, come back to earth as male. This is very unusual. Are you sure the baby is a girl?" he teased me, the midwife.

I wondered, "Gee, this man thinks it's not unusual to have two souls, but he think it's strange that two souls would incarnate in a female body! Go figure!"

Meanwhile Kak Mangku was explaining, "When two souls are in love, and they really want to be inseparable in the next life, they will incarnate like this, in one body. They must be *jodoh*, soul-mates, or it could not happen." Steve and I watched as he translated the Sanskrit letters out one by one, they spelled:

"S T E P H G R A C E S I T A. These are their names," Kak Mangku announced with confidence. "I'm sure you know them, they have reincarnated from your family line."

Steve took the wrinkled slip of paper and stared at it for a long time. Then tears began to well up in his eyes. "My grandparents were really in love. They died within a few days of each other. We used to joke they were still on their honeymoon to the last days. They were Stephen and Grace Sitz!"

Steve drew the lines between their names and Kak Mangku picked up the paper, "Hmmm, the A should have been a Z, but maybe their family name should have been Sita, like the wife of Rama. I am sorry, but sometimes there are small mistakes."

Adhiti's Placenta

In the cold winter of 1978, a tiny red headed girl was born into my hands. Adrian, a first time mother, was a university teacher in Iowa. Just before her baby was due, Adrian was informed that she could not have a homebirth where she lived on campus. Early on this snowy January morning, the college maintenance truck with a snow plough attached to the front fender delivered Adrian to my door. I was the only person she could think of to ask for help. As she stepped in from the howling snowstorm she said, "My midwives are caught in this blizzard. May I have my baby here?"

Because I had had my daughter at home, Adrian trusted me to help her; though I was only a twenty year old mom, with no experience, except for my own child's birth.

I assumed the midwives would arrive shortly, but baby Adhiti had something else in mind. I boiled water, not knowing what for. As Adrian labored, my two-year old daughter Déjà sat quietly, rubbing Adrian's back as her lovely baby girl emerged into the light of that lovely morning. It was a sweet gentle birth, and a wonderful portent that someday I would really be a midwife. We didn't even need the boiling water, except for tea!

Then Déjà ran downstairs to the kitchen and spontaneously brought up the very bowl her own placenta was caught in, just in time for the birth of the new baby's placenta. How did she know there was more to come after the birth? Somehow she did.

The ground was so frozen that Adhiti's father buried her placenta deep in the snow, in a plastic bowl. When Spring came the thaw revealed it, and the family gathered in the garden to give baby Adhiti's placenta a proper burial. In zthis way Adhiti's placenta found it's way into the Earth.

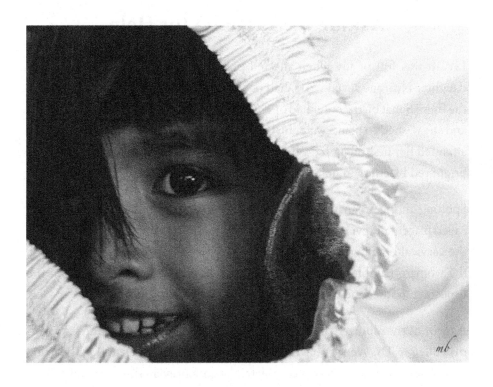

Several times over the years, parents have come to me repeatedly with a baby who has sniffles.

When I ask, "Where is the baby's placenta?"

They answer, "Oh it's still in the freezer. We haven't had time to give it a proper burial yet."

I advise them to get that placenta into the Earth Mother, where it will be warm and properly returned to the earth. After this, the baby's chronic colds clear completely!

Asking the Placenta for Help

LiWati was full of joy when she fell pregnant with her second baby. Her daughter Niti, age seven years, had been blissfully born at home. Since then, the Bumi Sehat birth center had opened just around the corner from her home, and she wished to plan a water birth there with the Bumi Sehat midwives who attended her first birth. However, her hopes and dreams were interrupted by bright red bleeding in her sixth week of pregnancy.

Spotting during pregnancy can be a symptom of a rare but dangerous condition called placenta previa: when the placenta lies so low in the uterus that it covers the cervical opening. If the placenta totally covers the opening of the cervix, the woman may bleed large amounts once dilation begins, putting both the expectant mother and the baby in danger.

As soon as she reported the bleeding, I took LiWati for an ultrasound scan with my colleague, Dr. Wedagama. It revealed that her baby's placenta was growing completely over her cervix, a complete placenta previa. This normally means that a cesarean birth is necessary. LiWati began to cry, she had so wanted to give birth naturally, without surgery. I suggested we all speak to the placenta: "Angel, please make your best effort to move up, away from the cervical opening, so that you and baby and mother may be safe." We also spoke to the baby: "Baby, you must communicate with your placenta angel and ask her to migrate north in your mom's uterus, so that you may be born naturally."

Dr. Wedagama gave me a confused look as we prayed to the placenta and baby. I know he was thinking that I was a bit crazy! "Well," he said doubtfully, "it would require a miracle, but what have we got to lose." He made a face so strange that LiWati actually laughed and wiped her tears. We sent her to bed rest for several weeks to relieve the stress on the cervix that was beginning to dilate due to the pressure of the placenta sitting on top of it. I also asked that we hold the vision and not disturb the placenta's concentration and best efforts to move up. Should there be no more incidents of bleeding, we would do no more ultrasound scans until LiWati was eight and a half months into her pregnancy.

After a few weeks of bed rest, LiWati slowly began to move around, but she was careful not to lift anything or to get fatigued. She balanced rest and activity with eating well, drinking plenty of clean water and taking organic Perfect Prenatal vitamin supplements donated by the wonderful people at New Chapter. She also continued speaking regularly to her baby's placenta. She talked and talked to her baby's placenta, asking it to make a safe path for her baby. I joined the discourse with the placenta, along with LiWati's family and the staff at the Bumi Sehat birth center. It became a village project to talk to LiWati's baby's placenta.

Two weeks before LiWati's due date, we showed up at Dr. Wedagama's office. He was sober, feeling like he and his ultrasound machine would be dark messengers. He wished so much that this young mother would not need a cesarean, but he knew that the odds were stacked up against natural childbirth for her. He was slower than usual getting set up. Finally, he applied the cold gel to LiWati's lovely belly and used the ultrasound wand to search inside, looking at the results of months of hope and faith.

As Dr. Wedagama searched first in the lower half of the uterus, we saw only the baby's head, perfectly positioned. But where was the placenta? He moved the wand up, higher and higher, then down, then up again. Finally way up north, as high as it could possibly be planted, there was our wonderful placenta! This baby's Angel had listened and had prevailed. LiWati would have the natural

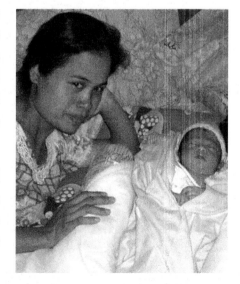

birth she prayed for. After jumping up and down for joy, Dr. Wedagama said, "Do you wish to know the sex of the baby?" LiWati said, "Oh no, this placenta and this baby need to be respected, I will wait until they come out to know if this is a baby boy or a girl. I am just so happy that I won't be needing a cesarean, thank you."

Three weeks later, Kadek Edi was born into a pool of flowers. When the placenta came, we floated him in a bowl in the tub and heaped beautiful flowers on top, thanking the baby's angel placenta for accomplishing a miracle.

Ari-Ari, The Healer

In1976, when Komang Bayu was only ten years old, he was taken home from the hospital, bloated and yellow, to die of hepatitis. This was customary in Bali, to bring the fatally ill home to die, to be close to the burial site of their *ari-ari*, their placentas.

When the family arrived home with the unconscious child he was in the final stages of dying. His grandfather took him in his arms and laid him on the earth, exactly where Bayu's placenta was buried. "*Ari-ari*," shouted the grandfather at the placenta, "take this child from his suffering now! If not... then heal him right now!"

Little Bayu opened his eyes, he sat up, he looked around, "May I have some food," he said. Within the hour the child had eaten and was up playing with his cousins.

Breastfeeding
So The Circle May Be Unbroken

Along with making meaningful rituals to honor our placentas, I believe that it is breastfeeding that maintains the circle of the mother-child continuum once the placental body is long gone. The evidence that breast milk is the optimum nourishment for babies is irrefutable. There is plenty of research proving that the benefits of breastfeeding are measurable into adulthood. The evidence that the breastfeeding relationship, driven by oxytocin, the hormone of love, is essential to maintaining the continuum of consciousness, is easy for most breastfeeding women to recognize. Nursing moms experience this continuum on a daily basis. A commonly told story:

"I went to the market, leaving my eight month old baby with her grandmother for a few minutes. Just as I was checking out, my milk came down without warning. This let me know without a doubt that my baby had awoken hungry and was calling me. I glanced at the clock and saw it was ten minutes before the hour. I rushed home to find my mother comforting my baby, who had indeed woke from her nap just at the moment my milk let down."

How do we explain this? Psychic phenomenon, or just life lived as it was meant to be? Breast feeding mothers will tell you, it is totally normal and natural to be linked psychically to their children. This link, as it grows strong, becomes compassion and connection with all beings. As women who have positive experiences of mothering grow into crones, they can nurture the world.

When one considers the benefits of breastfeeding, including improved health over a lifetime, improved intelligence, the psychological/spiritual benefits of being nourished in a way that naturally inspires a deep sense of security and self-esteem – well, it is tremendous. There is also the financial consideration: bottle-feeding is not only inferior to breastfeeding, but is so expensive that it often burdens young families, causing unnecessary stress. Add to that the costs of raising a bottle-fed child, who statistically will have more illnesses, allergies etc. and therefore greatly increased healthcare costs over a lifetime. In Indonesia, where I am a midwife, a bottle-fed baby is 300 times more likely to die in her first year of life than a breastfed baby.

The environmental impacts of feeding babies formula is profound. Consider the hectares of rainforest cleared everyday that will be allocated to cow pasture (approximately 1 hectare, 2.5 acres, are needed per cow). Methane from the off-gassing of bovine excrement and flatulents is a devastating contributor to global warming; Cattle produce 100 million tons of methane a year, 20% of the planet's total annual emmissions. It's not only the product itself, but the packaging and waste piling up in our dumps that must be factored in. From the box, packets and tins, to the plastic bottles and nipples, the inherant waste that further burdens the environment contributing to more tree loss, mineral extraction and depletion, and fossil fuel use and it's pollution, all in an attempt to produce a breast milk substitute to replace a 100% renewable, non-polluting, optimally healthy, psychologically and emotionally rewarding food source.

It would greatly benefit us as a society to reduce technological interventions in birth, to delay umbilical cord clamping and cutting, and to protect the natural bonding of mother and child. We must fiercely protect breastfeeding by raising the consciousness of health care givers: doctors, midwives, nurses, doulas, as well as family members, to believe in the natural birth process and breastfeeding. From this posturing we will be more effective in supporting breastfeeding start-up, and by protecting the foundation of each new human's ability to love, we can begin to heal birth, thereby healing our Earth.

Keeping placenta, cord and baby intact for as long as possible after the birth, protects the mother-child continuum by preventing separation, protecting breastfeeding.

Making Peace
for Lotus Birth

While speaking in Italy to a large group of Birth Keepers, I noticed that midwives and female nurses sat on one side of the hospital auditorium, obstetrical doctors and pediatricians sat on the other side.

The subject of delaying the clamping and cutting of the umbilical cords of babies became a heated argument. Midwives shouted, "They don't listen to us. They order us to cut the babies' cords, and we must obey or lose our jobs." OBGYN doctors protested, crying out, "The pediatricians are not cooperating with our requests for information!" Nurses complained, "The doctors don't listen to us either." The shouting became louder and louder.

Finally the microphone was handed to me. I waited until an uncomfortable silence fell upon the hall, then I asked, "When you speak to the doctors, are you loving them?"

"Of course not! They don't listen to us, we hate them" was the unanimous response to my question.

I waited again for silence in the hall. "Hmmm," I said, "When a person who hates me speaks, I must protect my heart, but that makes my ears close somehow and I cannot hear that person very well. When a person who is loving me speaks, I hear every word, loud and clearly."

Many Midwives and doctors, nurses and hospital administrators began to cry. Soon they were hugging one another. Dr. Giordano reports to me that now, at his hospital in Sicily, the staff is circulating literature on the benefits of delaying the clamping and cutting of babies' umbilical cords, and changes in protocol are being implemented.

Sometimes change, and peace, require that we simply ask the right question.

You Do Not Die Alone

The so called "natural fears": that of falling, loud sounds and the fear of pain or injury, are fears that are initiated at birth. Most humans adjust and learn to cope with these fears, as they are instinctive for all mammals and help us to survive. However, "unnatural fears": separation, abandonment, loneliness and death, are acquired due to trauma, and so, few of us ever overcome them.

We are not alone in the womb. From the beginning we enjoy the comfort of our placenta twin. This sister or brother sleeps and dreams and drums with us as we develop. With our placenta we share the lullaby of our mother's heartbeat. Indeed, we are not born alone, for the placenta shares our birth with us. Yet, due to modern birth protocols most of us are severed from this sacred twin prematurely and we learn to fear separation, abandonment and aloneness. This is birth trauma - original sin, if you will – and it is painful and may take a lifetime to heal, if at all.

If the indigenous Balinese belief has any truth to it, our placenta's body dies at birth in order to stay with us in spirit. This spirit brother or sister takes every earthly step with us. At the end of life, it helps us through the portal of death, just as it helped us navigate the portal into life, coming into the light just behind us, after guiding us through the birth canal. Once we are born, if the cord is not quickly severed, the placenta gives us her share of our blood, so that our brain, heart and all our organs are deeply enervated.

At death, our placenta appears beside us in spirit, now apparent to our "spirit" eyes. He or she accompanies us through the tunnel of light to the other side, and advocates for us. Just as the placenta advocated for your embryonic and fetal life, so too does it testify for you in the after-life. The placenta knows our life pattern and all the promises we made before coming into incarnation. Our own mothers do not even have this depth of soul knowledge about us.

Before the Gods, Goddesses, Saints, Angels, Seraphim and Cherubim, and all your departed relations, plus your relations soon to take reincarnation, your placenta will tell your life story. And you will see and feel and hear it all in detail, beginning from the last thing you heard in life and ending with the first word or sound you heard upon entering the world. This is why, as a midwife, I counsel parents to whisper an intentional word or message to the baby upon birth. Imagine a world in which each new baby receives a message of love, peace, trust and caring, to be carried by the soul. This sound, word, prayer, will take us higher when we recall, with the help of our placenta, our entire life story.

People often wish they could meet an angel. It is time we each remember and acknowledge the angel that helped us into the world and who is with us always. If you want to see the physical form of an angel, a miracle in the flesh, behold the placenta. Culture a friendship and kinship now with your placenta/guardian angel, and you may find that your life feels blessed. Later, when it is your time, you may be much more at ease when facing your own death. Call on him or her for help, anytime. Speak to your angel with your heart. Make small, meaningful rituals for him or her. By believing in your placenta/angel, you will learn to trust the dying process as a birth process into the next phase of your soul's life. I assure you, you were not born alone, and you will not die alone.

OM Shanti Shanti Shanti OM

Research to Consider

The following is a sampling of research on placenta's umbilical cords and the effects of the timing of late versus early cord clamping and cutting.

The Future: Our Beloved Placenta in Research

In the field of epigenetics, placentas may be the key in discovering the impact of environment, food, drink and even feelings on the genetic expression of human offspring. With the help of placentas scientists will be better able to diagnose, treat and even prevent disease and pathology.

Epigenetics in the Placenta, Matthew A. Maccani, B.A. and Carmen J. Marsit, Ph.D, *August 2009*

> "Important advances in placental epigenetics continue to elucidate a better understanding of the regulatory mechanisms of the placenta. Knowledge of such epigenetic mechanisms may be useful in identifying novel biomarkers for exposure, burden, or risk for disease. Such biomarkers may prove essential for developing new diagnostics for early diagnosis of risk factor and levels of exposure. Additionally, these aberrant patterns of miRNA expression, imprinting, DNA methylation, or histone modification may identify previously unknown pathways targeted for alteration, which, in turn, may serve as targets for novel drug treatment or prevention strategies. These epigenetic biomarkers can be brought from the bench top to the bedside and will be useful in helping clinicians better diagnose and prevent the onset of disease."

Studies Investigating the Benefits
of Delayed Cord Clamping & Cutting

Delayed cord clamping increases infants' iron stores, J. Mercer, D. Erickson-Owens, *The Lancet, Volume 367, Issue 9527, pp 1956-1958*

Neonatal prevention of iron deficiency: Placental transfusion is a cheap and physiological solution, Pisacane A, *BMJ, Jan 20, 1996. 312(7024):136-7*

"...estimated volume of placental transfusion varies from 20-60% of the existing blood volume (54-160 ml) depending on the time of clamping and the position in which the infant is held before clamping. Linderkamp and colleagues estimated that the amount of placental transfusion is 35 ml/kg of birth weight when term infants are kept at the level of the vaginal opening and the cord is clamped 3 minutes after birth. The same authors have recently investigated placing the neonate in the mother's abdomen and clamping the cord only once it stops pulsating. They found that these babies had blood volumes 32% higher than babies whose cords were clamped immediately after birth."

The early effects of delayed cord clamping in term infants born to Libyan mothers, Emhamed MO, van Rheenen P, *Brabin BJ. Trop Doct. Oct 2004, 34(4):218-22*

"Delaying cord clamping until the pulsations stop increases the red cell mass in term infants. It is a safe, simple and low cost delivery procedure that should be incorporated in integrated programmes aimed at reducing iron deficiency anaemia in infants in developing countries."

A study of the relationship between the delivery to cord clamping interval and the time of cord separation, *Oxford Midwives Research Group, Dec 7, 1991*

"There was an unexpectedly higher rate of breast feeding at home in the late clamped group which did reach statistical significance. Overall the trial provides no clear evidence for the benefit of early cord clamping."

The archived website www.cordclamping.com – The Dangerous Practice of Early Clamping of the Umbilical Cord – this is an extensive collection of writing pertaining to the subject of cord clamping. This site is striving to be the main web repository of scientific and medical support for allowing the baby to receive an optimal placental transfusion at the time of birth via an intact cord.

Late vs early clamping of the umbilical cord in full-term neonates: systematic review and meta-analysis of controlled trials, Hutton EK, Hassan ES, *JAMA. March 21, 2007. 297(11):1241-52*

> **Conclusions:** Delaying clamping of the umbilical cord in full-term neonates for a minimum of 2 minutes following birth is beneficial to the newborn, extending into infancy. Although there was an increase in polycythemia among infants in whom cord clamping was delayed, this condition appeared to be benign.

The effect of timing of cord clamping on neonatal venous hematocrit values and clinical outcome at term: a randomized, controlled trial, a study conducted by: Ceriani Cernadas JM, Carroli G, Pellegrini L, Otaño L, Ferreira M, Ricci C, Casas O, Giordano D, Lardizábal J of the Division of Neonatology Department of Pediatrics, Hospital Italiano de Buenos Aires, Buenos Aires, Argentina, *PEDIATRICS, the official Journal of the American Academy of Pediatrics,* Vol. 117 No. 4. April 2006

> **Background:** The umbilical cord is usually clamped immediately after birth. There is no sound evidence to support this approach, which might deprive the newborn of some benefits such as an increase in iron storage." The authors of this study went on to conclude that, "In term newborn infants, cord clamping at 1 or 3 minutes after birth resulted in an increase of venous hematocrit levels measured at 6 hours, within physiologic ranges, and a decreased prevalence of neonatal anemia without any harmful effect in newborns or mothers. Thus, this intervention seems to be safe and effective and could be implemented easily. The advantages of umbilical cord clamping at least at 1 minute after birth (remember, the medical 'normal' practice to IMMEDIATELY clamp and cut the umbilical cord) could decrease the prevalence of iron-deficiency anemia in the first year of life, especially in populations with limited access to health care. This trial was focused mainly on cord-clamping timing and its effect on the newborn, particularly in the first hours and days of life. We have shown our hypothesis to be true and additionally proved the protective effect of late cord clamping on neonatal anemia at birth."

The role of delayed umbilical cord clamping to control infant anaemia in resource-poor settings, Patrick van Rheenen, *2007*

> This is a good book – length compilation of scholarly studies on the benefits of Delayed Umbilical cord severance.

From a recent study at the University of Granada:

"...the clamping of the umbilical cord of newborns from full-term pregnancies, two minutes after the infant is expelled from the womb, makes no difference to hematocrit or hemoglobin levels of the umbilical cord vein compared to clamping the cord within 20 seconds. Thus, the study shows that early clamping (which is widely performed) is not justified."

Delayed clamping of the umbilical cord improves hematologic status of Guatemalan infants at 2 mo. of age, *Grajeda R et al, Am J Clin Nutr, 65:425-31, 1997*

Passive acquisition of protective antibodies reactive with Bordetella pertussis in newborns via placental transfer and breast-feeding, Quinello C, Quintilio W, Carneiro-Sampaio M, Palmeira P, *Department of Pediatrics, Faculdade de Medicina da Universidade de São Paulo, Brazil. Scand J Immunol. 72(1):66-73, July 2010*

This research highlights the importance of newborn acquisition of anti-pertussis antibodies: "Our data demonstrated the effectiveness of anti-pertussis antibodies in bacterial pathogenesis neutralization, emphasizing the importance of placental transfer and breast-feeding in protecting infants against respiratory infections caused by Bordetella pertussis."

Cardiopulmonary effects of placental transfusion, *Buckels Lj. J Pediatrics. (Supp 207):57-72, 1972*

"A large volume of placental blood is transferred to the newborn infant at delivery if the umbilical cord is left patent for some minutes. The significance of this transfusion in the immediate adaptation to extrauterine life is uncertain. To determine the physiologic consequences of placental transfusion, investigations were made during the first hours of life on 15 full-term infants whose cords were clamped immediately, and on 17 whose cords were clamped 5 minutes after birth. Infants with immediate cord clamping had anemia, hypotension, and acidosis comparable to those with delayed cord clamping. These infants also had heart murmurs, not heard when cord clamping was delayed."

Lotus Birth: A Ritual for our Times, Sarah J. Buckley, 2000

Zoonomia: The Laws of Organic Life (2nd ed.), Darwin, E. London: *J. Johnson, 1796*

Early Childhood anemia and mild to moderate mental retardation,
Hurtado EK et al. *Am J Clin Nut. 69 (1): 115-119, 1999*

> **Results:** "Logistic regression showed an increased likelihood of mild or moderate mental retardation associated with anemia,"

> I include this study to highlight the dangers of newborn anemia and the causal relationship, to wit, many studies show that delaying the ligation of the umbilical cord reduces the incidence of newborn anemia.

Early Clamping of the Umbilical Cord: Cutting the Ties that Bind, Mermer, Cory A, *Potential Dangers of Childbirth Interventions, The Examiner of Medical Alternatives, pp 74-78, April 2000*

How the Cord Clamp Injures Your Baby's Brain, Morley, M.B., George M., *Ch.B., FACOG. Cordclamping.com, Feb 26, 2002*

Cord Closure: Can Hasty Cord Clamping Injure the Newborn?, Morley M. *OBG Management. pp 29-36, July 1998*

Effect of gravity on placental transfusion, Yao AC, Lind J. *Lancet. ii: 505-8, 1969*

Placental transfusion, Yao AC, Lind J. *AM J dis Child. 127: 128-141, 1974*

Distribution of blood between infant and placenta after birth, Yao AC et al. *Lancet. ii: 871-873, 1969*

> This discussion has been going on a long time, evidence this study: *Pediatrics* Vol. 40 No. 1. July 1967. pp 109-126

Placental Transfusion: Early Versus Late Clamping of the Umbilical Cord, Arthur J. Moss M.D., Michelle Monset-Couchard M.D, *The Division of Cardiology, Department of Pediatrics, UCLA School of Medicine, California*

> IATROGENIC interruption of the placental circulation at birth has, in most cases become an automatic procedure with little or no regard for the physiologic alterations evoked or for their subsequent effect upon the fetus. The relative merits of "early" and "late" clamping of the umbilical cord have been the subject of controversy for many years. More recently it has been suggested that the time of cord clamping may be involved in the pathogenesis of idiopathic respiratory distress syndrome (IRDS). As of this writing, the controversy of "early" versus "late" clamping remains unsettled.

Review of the pertinent literature indicates that this is due largely to failure to define uniformly "early" and "late," failure by many to consider the effects of onset of respiration, of gravity, of uterine contractions, and, in some instances, to conclusions not completely warranted by supporting data.

In view of the potential significance of the issue and the current confusion surrounding it, critical re-examination appears to be in order. A major purpose of this review is to call attention to the areas of investigation needing further documentation.

Effect on Blood Volume

The blood volume of newborn infants has been studied by a number of investigators.

Effect of Leboyer childbirth on cardiac output, cerebral and gastrointestinal blood flow velocities in full-term neonates, Nelle M et al. *AM J Perinatol, 12:212-6, 1995*

Placental transfusion advantage and disadvantage, Peltonen T. *Eur J Pediatr. 137:141-146, 1981*

Neonatal prevention of iron deficiency. Placental transfusion is a cheap and physiological solution, Pisacane A. *British Medical Journal, 312:136-7, 1996*

Late umbilical cord-clamping as an intervention for reducing iron deficiency anaemia in term infants in developing and industrialised countries: a systematic review, Van Rheenen P, Brabin BJ, *Ann Trop Paediatr, 2004*

Maternal effects of early and late clamping of the umbilical cord, Walsh, S., *The Lancet: 997, May 11, 1968*

Abstract Duration of the third stage of labour, and incidence of retained placental secundines and post-partum bleeding were investigated in fifty-nine mothers of early-clamped infants and in fifty-eight mothers of late-clamped infants. Post-partum bleeding was significantly greater in mothers of early-clamped infants and was unrelated to such factors as overdistension of the uterus, medication, and soft-tissue injury. No difference in duration of the third stage of labour was found. Manual removal of placental secundines was required in five mothers of early-clamped infants, an incidence of 9%.

The roles and vital importance of placental blood to the newborn infant, Wardrop CA, Holland BM. *J Perinat Med. 23 :139 –143, 1995*

Studies Concerning Premature Infants

Delayed cord clamping in preterm infants delivered at 34–36 weeks' gestation: a randomised controlled trial, C A Ultee1, J van der Deure1, J Swart2, C Lasham3, A L van Baar4, *Department of Paediatrics, Deventer Hospital, The Netherlands 2 Wilhelmina Children's Hospital, Utrecht, The Netherlands 3 Department of Paediatrics, Hospital Gooi-Noord, The Netherlands 4 Paediatric Psychology, Tilburg University, The Netherlands. Correspondence to: Dr C A Ultee, Department of Paediatrics, Deventer Hospital, Postbus 5001 fesevurstraat, Deventer 7400 GC, The Netherlands*

Background: "Even mild iron deficiency and anaemia in infancy may be associated with cognitive deficits. A delay in clamping the cord improves haematocrit levels and results in greater vascular stability and less need for packed cell transfusions for anaemia in the first period after birth. Follow-up data on haemoglobin levels after the neonatal period were not available."

Objective: "To provide neonatal and follow-up data for the effects of early or delayed clamping of the cord."

Methods: "37 premature infants (gestational age 34 weeks, 0 days–36 weeks, 6 days) were randomly assigned to one of two groups in the first hour after birth, and at 10 weeks of age. In one group the umbilical cord was clamped within 30 seconds (mean (SD) 13.4 (5.6)) and in the other, it was clamped at 3 minutes after delivery. In the neonatal period blood glucose and haemoglobin levels were determined. At 10 weeks of age haemoglobin and ferritin levels were determined."

Results: "The late cord-clamped group showed consistently higher haemoglobin levels than the early cord-clamped group, both at the age of 1 hour (mean (SD) 13.4 (1.9) mmol/l vs 11.1 (1.7) mmol/l), and at 10 weeks (6.7 (0.75) mmol/l vs 6.0 (0.65) mmol/l). No relationship between delayed clamping of the umbilical cord and pathological jaundice or polycythaemia was found."

Conclusion: "Immediate clamping of the umbilical cord should be discouraged."

Delayed Cord Clamping in Very Preterm Infants Reduces the Incidence of Intraventricular Hemorrhage and Late-Onset Sepsis: A Randomized, Controlled Trial, *Author manuscript; available in PMC,* Judith S. Mercer, DNSc, CNM,a Betty R. Vohr, MD,b Margaret M. McGrath, DNSc,a James F. Padbury, MD,b Michael Wallach, MD,b and William Oh, *MDb Pediatrics, September 14, 2006*

Umbilical cord clamping and preterm infants: a randomized trial, Kinmond S et al. *British Medical Journal, 306: 172-175, 1993*

Delay in Cutting the Cord Helps Premature Babies, Levin, Aaron, Pediatrics, *2012 Mar;129(3):e667-72. doi: 10.1542/peds. 2011-2550. Epub 2012 Feb 13, Oct 18, 2004*

Hemodynamic effects of delayed cord clamping in premature infants, Sommers R, Stonestreet BS, Oh W, Laptook A, Yanowitz TD, Raker C, Mercer J.

Source: Department of Neonatology, Women & Infants Hospital of Rhode Island & Alpert Medical School of Brown University, Providence, RI 02905, USA

Background and Objective: Delayed cord clamping (DCC) has been advocated during preterm delivery to improve hemodynamic stability during the early neonatal period. The hemodynamic effects of DCC in premature infants after birth have not been previously examined. Our objective was to compare the hemodynamic differences between premature infants randomized to either DCC or immediate cord clamping (ICC).

Methods: This prospective study was conducted on a subset of infants who were enrolled in a randomized controlled trial to evaluate the effects of DCC versus ICC. Entry criteria included gestational ages of 24(0) to 31(6) weeks. Twins and infants of mothers with substance abuse were excluded. Serial Doppler studies were performed at 6 ± 2, 24 ± 4, 48 ± 6, and 108 ± 12 hours of life. Measurements included superior vena cava blood flow, right ventricle output, middle cerebral artery blood flow velocity (BFV), superior mesenteric artery BFV, left ventricle shortening fraction, and presence of a persistent ductus arteriosus.

Results: Twenty-five infants were enrolled in the DCC group and 26 in the ICC group. Gestational age, birth weight, and male gender were similar. Admission laboratory and clinical events were also similar. DCC resulted in significantly higher superior vena cava blood flow over the study period, as well as greater right ventricle output and right ventricular stroke volumes at 48 hours. No differences were noted in middle cerebral artery BFV, mean superior mesenteric artery BFV, shortening fraction, or the incidence of a persistent ductus arteriosus.

Conclusion: DCC in premature infants is associated with potentially beneficial hemodynamic changes over the first days of life.

Stem Cell/Umbilical Cord Blood Banking

Letter: Commercial cord blood banking Immediate cord clamping is not safe, David J R Hutchon, consultant obstetrician and gynaecologist Memorial Hospital, Darlington

EDITOR—Edozien has provided a balanced analysis of the issue of commercial cord banking. 1 A need exists for further emphasis on the importance of delayed cord clamping. In addition to the Cochrane meta-analysis; 2 further trials have shown substantial benefits in very low birthweight infants; 3 and also term infants. Cord blood collection must not be allowed to restrict this practice. The value of delayed cord clamping has been shown whereas the value of commercial cord blood banking is still largely hypothetical at present.

Commercial cord blood banking is an insurance, not with a monetary return in the event of a claim but with the prospect of a successful medical treatment. Like all commercial insurance there is a premium to pay and risk of collapse unless the venture is underwritten by the government or the insurance industry as a whole.

References:

1. Edozien LC. *NHS maternity units should not encourage commercial banking of umbilical cord blood.* BMJ 2006;333: 801-4. http://bmj.bmjjournals.com/cgi/ijlink?linkType=FULL&journalCode=bmj&resid=333/7572/801

2. Rabe H, Reynolds G, Diaz-Rossello J. *Early versus delayed umbilical cord clamping in preterm infants.* 2004. Cochrane Database Syst Rev. (4):CD003248.

3. Mercer JS, Vohr, BR, McGrath MM, Padbury JF, Wallach M, Oh W. *Delayed cord clamping in very preterm infants reduces the incidence of intraventricular hemorrhage and late-onset sepsis: a randomized, controlled trial.* 2006. Pediatrics. 117: 1235-42.

Cord Blood Banking for Potential Future Transplantation, *The American Academy of Pediatrics, Jan 1, 2007:* "A number of private for-profit companies have been established that encourage parents to bank their children's cord blood for their own autologous use or for directed donor allogeneic use for a family member should the need arise. Parents have been encouraged to bank their infants' cord blood as a form of "biological insurance." Physicians, employees, and/or consultants of such companies may have potential conflicts of interest in recruiting patients because of their own financial gain. Annual disclosure of the financial interest and potential conflicts of interest must be made to institutional review boards that are charged with the responsibility of mitigation of these disclosures and risks. Families may be vulnerable to the emotional effects of marketing for cord blood banking at the time of birth of a child and may look to their physicians for advice. No accurate estimates exist of the likelihood of children to need their own stored cord blood stem cells in the future. The range of available estimates is from 1 in 1000 to more than 1 in 200,000. The potential for children needing their own cord blood stem cells for future autologous use is controversial presently. There also is no evidence of the safety or effectiveness of autologous cord blood stem cell transplantation for the treatment of malignant neoplasms. Indeed, there is evidence demonstrating the presence of DNA mutations in cord blood obtained from children who subsequently develop leukemia. Thus, an autologous cord blood transplantation might even be contraindicated in the treatment of a child who develops leukemia."

Stem Cell Banking controversy, *Science Daily, March 6, 2008.* Solving a long-standing biological mystery, UCLA stem cell researchers have discovered that blood stem cells, the cells that later differentiate into all the cells in the blood supply, originate and are nurtured in the placenta.

"It was a big mystery, where these cells originated," said Mikkola, an assistant professor of molecular, cell and developmental biology. "This is the first time we can really say definitively that blood stem cells are generated in the placenta. There's no more speculation."

"Using this model, we identified that the placenta has the potential to make hematopoietic (blood) stem cells with full differentiation ability to create all the major lineages of blood cells," Mikkola said. "The placenta acts as a sort of kindergarten for these newly made blood stem cells, giving them the first education they need."

This Study suggests we just allow the natural transfusion of placental blood to the baby!

Mankind's first natural stem cell transplant, Jose N. Tolosa, Dong-Hyuk Park, David J. Eve, Stephen K. Klasko, Cesario V. Borlongan, Paul R. Sanberg, *2010 Journal of Cellular and Molecular Medicine*

Studies that Concern Rh-Sensitization

Management of the Third Stage of Labor with particular reference to reduction of feto-maternal transfusion, *Lapido, O. BMJ 1 : 721-3, 1972*

"Rh-sensitization and Third Stage of Labour SIR,-Mr. 0. A. Ladipo (18 March 1972, p. 721) draws attention to the possibility that rhesus sensitization is to some extent an iatrogenic phenomenon. By interference with nature's management of the third stage of labour, particularly by early clamping of the placental end of the severed cord, it could be that doctors and midwives cause more potentially sensitizing fetal cells to enter the maternal circulation."

This study also includes a table demonstrating higher APGAR scores for the newborns in the late cord clamping/cutting group.

Placental drainage and feto-maternal transfusion, Moncrieff D et al. *Lancet.* *2:453, 1986*

This study was conducted upon cesarean mothers and points to the fact that allowing the baby's blood to flow freely to the baby, reduces the incidence of Rh sensitization in Rh− mothers.

Placental drainage and feto-maternal transfusion, C Moncrieff D et al, *Lancet,* *2:453, 1986*

"The timing of cord clamping may have effects on both mother and infant. Early cord clamping should be avoided in rhesus negative women as it increases the risk of feto-maternal transfusion. However, allowing free bleeding from the placental end of the cord reduces this risk. [i] Delayed cord clamping results in a shift of blood from the placenta to the infant. The volume transfused varies between 20% and 50% of neonatal blood volume, depending on when the cord is clamped and at what level the baby is held prior to clamping. [ii] There have been concerns that the increase in the newborn's blood volume and red blood cell volume that is associated with delayed cord clamping could result in overload of the heart and respiratory difficulties. These effects have not, however, been demonstrated. Placental transfusion associated with delayed cord clamping provides additional iron to the infant's reserves and may reduce the frequency of iron-deficiency anaemia later in infancy. [iii] Early cord clamping reduces the extent of placental transfusion to the baby and results in significantly lower haematocrit and haemoglobin levels in newborns. [v]"

Studies Concerning Tetanus

Maternal and neonatal tetanus, Roper MH, Vandelaer JH, Gasse FL. *Lancet. 370: 1947-1959, 2007*

Michel Odent, *The Lancet 2008, Volume: 371, Issue 9610. pp 385-386*

Studies Concerning Food Manipulation: Hybrids and GMO

Glyphosate Formulations Induce Apoptosis and Necrosis in Human Umbilical, Embryonic, and Placental Cells, Nora Benachour, Gilles-Eric Séralini, *Chem. Res. Toxicol, December 23, 2008*

Genetically Modified Soy Linked to Sterility, Infant Mortality in Hamsters, Jeffrey M. Smith, *Consumerism, GMOs, Health & Disease, May 4, 2010*

Maternal Mortality in Bali, Indonesia, Dr. Inne Susante, Dr I.B. Asawa and Judith A. Fortney Ph.D

Reduction of Maternal Mortality, a joint WHO/UNICEF/World Bank Statement 1999, WHO Geneva

---

Compilation of additional Research in Delayed versus Immediate Clamping and Cutting of Babies' Umbilical Cords

Parents and health providers all wish for the same thing, optimal health, intelligence and longevity for the mothers and babies in their care. The following is a review of the more current research on the effects of delayed versus immediate clamping and cutting of babies' umbilical cords.

Effect of delayed versus early umbilical cord clamping on neonatal outcomes and iron status at 4 months: a randomised controlled trial, *MJ 2011;343:d7157 doi: 10.1136/bmj.d7157 (Published 15 November 2011)*

Conclusions and policy implications: We conclude that delayed cord clamping, in this randomised controlled trial, resulted in improved ferritin levels and reduced the prevalence of iron deficiency at 4 months of age. Delayed clamping also reduced the prevalence of neonatal anaemia at 2 days of age without increasing the rate of respiratory symptoms or need for phototherapy in this sample of 382 full term infants born in a high income country. Two meta-analyses of clamping studies performed in low or middle income countries with a high general prevalence of anaemia found similar effects on ferritin as we did and concluded that this effect is clinically relevant and should lead to a change in practice. Iron deficiency even without anaemia has been associated with impaired development among infants. Our results suggest that delayed cord clamping also benefits infant health in regions with a relatively low prevalence of iron deficiency and should be considered as standard care for full term deliveries after uncomplicated pregnancies. Further studies are needed to explore long term health effects of delayed and early cord clamping.

…Our results therefore strongly suggest that delayed cord clamping is not associated with any increase in the need of phototherapy in term infants, in agreement with the recent meta-analysis in JAMA.

Timing of umbilical cord-clamping and infant anaemia: the role of maternal anaemia.

Conclusion: The study contributes additional evidence in support of delayed cord-clamping. This intervention is likely to have the most public health impact in areas with a high prevalence of anaemia during pregnancy.

Effect of timing of umbilical cord clamping of term infants on maternal and neonatal outcomes (Review). McDonald SJ, Middleton P, Dowswell T, Morris PS. *Editorial group: Cochrane Pregnancy and Childbirth Group.*

Publication status and date: New search for studies and content updated (conclusions changed), published in Issue 7, 2013. Review content assessed as up-to-date: 14 March 2013.

Authors' conclusions: A more liberal approach to delaying clamping of the umbilical cord in healthy term infants appears to be warranted, particularly in light of growing evidence that delayed cord clamping increases early haemoglobin concentrations and iron stores in infants. Delayed cord clamping is likely to be beneficial as long as access to treatment for jaundice requiring phototherapy is available.

Plain Language Summary: Effect of timing of umbilical cord clamping of term infants on mother and baby outcomes.
At the time of birth, the infant is still attached to the mother via the umbilical cord, which is part of the placenta. The infant is usually separated from the placenta by clamping the cord. This clamping is one part of the third stage of labour (the time from birth of the baby until delivery of the placenta) and the timing can vary according to clinical policy and practice. Although early cord clamping has been thought to reduce the risk of bleeding after birth (postpartum haemorrhage), this review of 15 randomised trials involving a total of 3911 women and infant pairs showed no significant difference in postpartum haemorrhage rates when early and late cord clamping (generally between one and three minutes) were compared. There were, however, some potentially important advantages of delayed cord clamping in healthy term infants, such as higher birthweight, early haemoglobin concentration, and increased iron reserves up to six months after birth. These need to be balanced against a small additional risk of jaundice in newborns that requires phototherapy.

Discussion: The importance of delayed cord clamping for Aboriginal babies: A life-enhancing advantage. *Rosemary Weckert, Heather Hancock*

Summary: Third stage management has typically focused on women and postpartum haemorrhage. Clamping and cutting the umbilical cord following the birth of the baby has continued to be a routine part of this focus. Active versus physiological management of third stage is generally accepted as an evidence-based plan for women to avoid excessive blood loss. Other considerations around this decision are rarely considered, including the baby's perspective. This paper provides a review of the literature regarding timing of clamping and cutting of the umbilical cord and related issues, and discusses the consequences for babies and in particular Aboriginal babies. Iron stores in babies are improved (among other important advantages) if the cord is left to stop pulsating for 3 min before being clamped. Such a simple measure of patience and informed practice can make a long lasting difference to a baby's health and for Aboriginal babies this advantage can be critical in the short and the long term for their development and wellbeing. To achieve much needed reductions in infancy anaemia and essential increases in infant survival, delayed cord clamping and cutting is recommended for all Aboriginal babies.

Conclusion: Clamping and cutting of the umbilical cord at 3 min following birth (including the need for resuscitation which can be conducted with the baby between the mother's legs while the cord is still patent and attached) is a safe option for optimal placental transfusion regardless of the baby's weight. This practice is completely cost effective (in the immediate and longer term) non-intervening and not harmful for mother or baby. An oxytocic could be administered if necessary to decrease maternal blood loss without needing to clamp and cut the cord. Every baby, and most importantly every Aboriginal baby, regardless of their gestation should have the right and significant advantages of their cord being clamped and cut 3 min after their birth to achieve much needed reductions in infancy anaemia and essential increases in infant survival. Such a simple measure of patience and informed practice with such life enhancing advantages for all babies, especially Aboriginal babies, is vital. Keeping the cord patent and extending the time before cord clamping and cutting for at least several minutes after the birth of the baby, or preferably until cord pulsations cease, is recommended for all Aboriginal babies as an effective primary health strategy by midwives and doctors.

Clinical Rounds: Delayed Clamping of the Umbilical Cord: A Review With Implications for Practice,Gina Eichenbaum-Pikser, CNM, MSN and Joanna S. Zasloff, CNM, MSN

Discussion: It has been postulated that delayed cord clamping may increase rates of hyperbilirubinemia, polycythemia, and transient tachypnea in the newborn or maternal hemorrhage. However, delayed cord clamping has never been proven to increase the rate of neonatal symptomatic disease or maternal blood loss.

Implications for clinical practice: The practice of delayed cord clamping has shown many benefits to the newborn with no documentation of significant risk. As such, it is incumbent upon clinicians to educate their clients about the physiologic impact of the practice of delayed cord clamping and to involve women in this decision, as we do in so many other clinical scenarios.

Effect of delayed versus early umbilical cord clamping on neonatal outcomes and iron status at 4 months: a randomised controlled trial, Andersson O, Hellström-Westas L, Andersson D, Domellöf M, *BMJ. 2011 Nov 15;343:d7157. doi: 10.1136/bmj.d7157*, **Source:** Department of Paediatrics, Hospital of Halland, Halmstad, SE-301 85 Halmstad, Sweden

Effects of delayed compared with early umbilical cord clamping on maternal postpartum hemorrhage and cord blood gas sampling: a randomized trial, Andersson O, Hellström-Westas L, Andersson D, Clausen J, Domellöf M, *Acta Obstet Gynecol Scand. 2013 May;92(5):567-74. doi: 10.1111/j.1600-0412.2012.01530.x. Epub 2012 Oct 17*, **Source:** Department of Pediatrics, Hospital of Halland, Halmstad Department of Women's and Children's Health, Uppsala University, Uppsala, Sweden.

Conclusions: Delayed cord clamping, compared with early, did not have a significant effect on maternal postpartum hemorrhage or on the proportion of valid blood gas samples. We conclude that delayed cord clamping is a feasible method from an obstetric perspective.

Delayed cord clamping and haemoglobin levels in infancy: a randomised controlled trial in term babies, van Rheenen P, de Moor L, Eschbach S, de Grooth H, Brabin B, *Trop Med Int Health. 2007 May;12(5):603-16*, **Source:** Department of Paediatrics, Paediatric Gastroenterology, University Medical Centre, Groningen, The Netherlands

Long-term brain and behavioral consequences of early iron deficiency, Georgieff MK, *Nutr Rev. 2011 Nov;69 Suppl 1:S43-8. doi: 10.1111/j.1753-4887.2011.00432.x*, **Source:** Center for Neurobehavioral Development, University of Minnesota School of Medicine and College of Education and Human Development, Minneapolis, Minnesota, USA

Early iron deficiency not only affects brain and behavioral function during the period of iron deficiency, it persists long after treatment. The mechanisms include long-term alterations in dopamine metabolism, myelination, and hippocampal structure and function. Recent studies have demonstrated long-term genomic changes, which suggests the regulation of brain function is fundamentally altered.

Delayed Umbilical Cord Clamping in Premature Neonates. Joseph W. Kaempf, MD, Mark W. Tomlinson, MD, Andrew J. Kaempf, BS, YingXing Wu, MD, Lian Wang, MS, Nicole Tipping, RN, and Gary Grunkemeier, PhD

Results: In VLBW neonates (77 delayed umbilical cord clamping, birth weight [mean standard deviation] 1,099 266 g; 77 early umbilical cord clamping 1,058 289 g), delayed umbilical cord clamping was associated with less delivery room resuscitation, higher Apgar scores at 1 minute, and higher hematocrit. Delayed umbilical cord clamping was not associated with significant differences in the overall transfusion rate, peak bilirubin, any of the principle Vermont Oxford Network outcomes, or mortality. In LBW neonates (172 delayed umbilical cord clamping, birth weight [mean standard deviation] 2,159 384 g; 172 early umbilical cord clamping 2,203 447 g), delayed umbilical cord clamping was associated with higher hematocrit and was not associated with a change in delivery room resuscitation or Apgar scores or with changes in the transfusion rate or peak bilirubin. Regression analysis showed increasing gestational age and birth weight and delayed umbilical cord clamping were the best predictors of higher hematocrit and less delivery room resuscitation.

Conclusion: Delayed umbilical cord clamping can safely be performed in singleton premature neonates and is associated with a higher hematocrit, less delivery room resuscitation, and no significant changes in neonatal morbidities.

Rethinking Placental Transfusion and Cord Clamping Issues, Debra A. Erickson-Owens, PhD, CNM, J Perinat Neonat Nurs r Vo 2012. Judith S. Mercer, PhD, CNM, FACNM

Physiologic effects of placental transfusion on the infant: When cord clamping is delayed at birth or the cord is milked, infants experience placental transfusion as whole blood is transferred (or transfused) from the placenta to the infant during the first few minutes of life. This blood contains not only volume and red blood cells but also millions of stem cells important in repairing tissue and building immunocompetence. The red blood cells are a major source of iron during the first few months of life. When the cord is cut rapidly, the infant has no access to approximately 30 mL/kg (of birth weight) of blood—about 30% of the fetal-placental blood volume. Placental transfusion facilitates an increase in the circulatory bed at the same time that the infant's various organs (lung, liver, kidney, etc) assume the many functions maintained by the placenta during fetal life. This additional blood volume may reduce the vulnerability of infants to inflammatory processes and provide protection against infection.

Fetal and neonatal blood volume: Throughout pregnancy, blood flows in a continuous circuit from fetus to placenta (via the 2 umbilical arteries) and back to fetus (via the 1 umbilical vein). The fetal heart is the driver for this process, contracting with enough force to perfuse the most distant placental villi. The amount of whole blood in the fetal-placental circulation is estimated to be 110 to 115 mL/kg of fetal weight throughout gestation. During fetal life, the blood flow to the lungs is only 10% of the fetal cardiac output. The placenta is the organ of respiration and it adequately oxygenates the fetus with more than 50% of the fetal cardiac output circulating through it at any one time. At birth, the cardiac output to the lungs must rapidly change from 10% to 45%–55% to adapt to air respiration in the newborn lungs. Delayed cord clamping delivers the volume of blood needed for this adaptation. The circulation in the cord continues for several minutes after birth and placental transfusion results in approximately 30% more blood volume compared with infants with ICC.

Timing of umbilical cord clamping after birth for optimizing placental transfusion, *Tonse N.K. Raju Volume 25, Number 2, April 2013*

Clamping, Ryan M. McAdams, *MD Obstetrics & Gynecology Vol. 123, No. 3, March 2014*

Umbilical cord clamping after birth - Better not to rush, Andrew Weeks, senior lecturer in obstetrics School of Reproductive and Developmental Medicine, University of Liverpool, Liverpool L8 7SS

Current best evidence: a review of the literature on umbilical cord clamping, Mercer JS. *J Midwifery Womens Health. 2001 Nov-Dec;46(6):402-14*

Delayed cord clamping increases infants' iron stores. *Mercer J, Erickson-Owens D. Lancet. 2006 Jun 17;367(9527):1956-8*

Neonatal transitional physiology: a new paradigm. *Mercer JS, Skovgaard RL. J Perinat Neonatal Nurs 2002 Mar;15(4):56-75*

Early clamping of the umbilical cord at birth, a practice developed without adequate evidence, causes neonatal blood volume to vary 25% to 40%. Such a massive change occurs at no other time in one's life without serious consequences, even death. Early cord clamping may impede a successful transition and contribute to hypovolemic and hypoxic damage in vulnerable newborns. The authors present a model for neonatal transition based on and driven by adequate blood volume rather than by respiratory effort to demonstrate how neonatal transition most likely occurs at a normal physiologic birth.

Endnotes

Introduction

1. World Health Organization Reproductive Health Publications. *Timing of Cord Clamping*. Care in Normal Birth: A Practical Guide Report, section 5.5.

What is the Placenta?

1. Vanessa E. Murphy, Roger Smith, Warwick B. Giles and Vicki L. Clifton (2006). *Endocrine Regulation of Human Fetal Growth: The Role of the Mother, Placenta, and Fetus*. The Endocrine Society.

2. Vanessa E. Murphy, Roger Smith, Warwick B. Giles and Vicki L. Clifton (2006). *Endocrine Regulation of Human Fetal Growth: The Role of the Mother, Placenta, and Fetus*. The Endocrine Society.

3. Bowen R (2000-08-06). *Placental Hormones*. Retrieved 2008-03-12.

4. Harun Yahya. *Placenta the bridge of Life*.

5. Robert K. Creasy, Robert Resnik, Jay D. Iams (September 2003). *Maternal-Fetal Medicine: Principles and Practice*. pp 31-32. ISBN 9780721600048.

6. The 'Jeeva' Project: *Investigating the Indigenous Practice of Reviving the Lifeless Newborn by Stimulation of the Placenta*. A Concept Note for a Project Proposal (July 2007).

7. Mira Sadgopal (April 18, 2009). *Can maternity services open up to the indigenous traditions of midwifery?* Economic & Political Weekly EPW vol xliv no 16.

Placenta: Our Hero/Heroine in Myth and History

1. Gorgon. Retrieved from Wikipedia: http://en.wikipedia.org/wiki/Gorgon

2. Egyptology. Retrieved from Wikipedia: http://en.wikipedia.org/wiki/Egyptology

3. Taurt. In Encyclopædia Britannica online. Retrieved from: www.britannica.com/EBchecked/topic/584405/Taurt

4. Taurt. In Encyclopædia Britannica online. Retrieved from: www.britannica.com/EBchecked/topic/584405/Taurt

5. Clyde E. Keeler (1960). *Secrets of the Cuna Earth Mother: A Comparative Study of Ancient Religions*. Exposition Press. pp 53.

6. Clyde E. Keeler (1960). *Secrets of the Cuna Earth Mother: A Comparative Study of Ancient Religions*. Exposition Press. pp 54.

7. Clyde E. Keeler (1960). *Secrets of the Cuna Earth Mother: A Comparative Study of Ancient Religions.* Exposition Press. pp 273.

8. Clyde E. Keeler (1960). *Secrets of the Cuna Earth Mother: A Comparative Study of Ancient Religions.* Exposition Press. pp 68.

9. Clyde E. Keeler (1960). *Secrets of the Cuna Earth Mother: A Comparative Study of Ancient Religions.* Exposition Press. pp 78.

10. L. De Mause, Foundations of Psychohistory (New York: Creative Roots, 1982): 289. E. Noble, *Primal Connections: How Our Experiences from Conception to Birth Influence Our Emotions, Behavior and Health.* New York: Fireside, Simon & Schuster, 1993): 83.

11. Leavitt, Judith Walzer (1986). *Brought to Bed: Childbearing in America, 1750 to 1950.* New York: Oxford University Press. pp 21-37.

12. *Akhet the Horizon, Women in Ancient Egypt.* Ancient Egyptian Relition. Retrieved from: www.philae.nu/akhet/Childbirth.html

13. Victor Montejo. *The Elders Dreamed of Fire Religion and Repression in the Guatemalan Highlands.*

14. Ministry of Justice New Zealand (2001). *He Hinatore ki te Ao Maori: A Glimpse into the Maori World: Maori Perspectives on Justice.* Wellington, NZ: Crown Copyright.

15. O. Boryak (Spring 2003). *The Midwife in Traditional Ukrainian Culture: Ritual, Folklore and Mythology.* Midwifery Today 65: 53.

16. Republic of Turkey Ministry of Culture and Tourism (2004). *Traditions to Do with Birth.* Retrieved from: www.kultur.gov.tr/EN

17. J. Quintner (26 November, 1999). *Taking the Cake.* Medical Observer (Australia) 65.

18. J. Quintner (26 November, 1999). *Taking the Cake.* Medical Observer (Australia) 65.

19. Fred B. Eiseman Jr. *Bali, Sekala and Niskala, Vol. 1: Essays on Religion, Ritual, and Art.*

20. Creation Myth. Retrieved from Wikipedia: http://en.wikipedia.org/wiki/Creation_Myth

21. Clyde E. Keeler (1960). *Secrets of the Cuna Earth Mother: A Comparative Study of Ancient Religions.* Exposition Press. pp 36.

22. Clyde E. Keeler (1960). *Secrets of the Cuna Earth Mother: A Comparative Study of Ancient Religions.* Exposition Press. pp 49.

23. Paul Bahn (May/June 1991). Excerpt from the article *Mystery of the Placenta Pots.* Archaeology Magazine. pp 18-19.

24. Bernard Faure, Kao Professor in Japanese Religion. *The Watchful Twins: Gods and Destiny in East Asian Buddhism* [Lecture]. Columbia University.

25. Edie Farwell and Anne Hubbell Maiden (Spring 1992). *The Wisdom Of Tibetan Childbirth.* In Context #31, Context Institute. pp 26.

Modern Treatment of the Placenta

1. Patricia Guthrie (July 7, 1999). *Many Cultures Revere Placenta, By Product of Childbirth.* Cox News Service.

2. George M. Morley, M.B., Ch. B., FACOG (February 21, 2002). *How the Cord Clamp Injures Your Baby's Brain.*

3. George M. Morley (April 11, 2002). *Why Do Babies Cry? The Anatomical and Physiological Changes During the Moments After Birth.*

4. Tetanus. World Health Orgnaization (updated 13 February, 2008). Retrieved from: www.who.int/immunization/topics/tetanus/en/

5. Roper MH, Vandelaer JH, Gasse FL (2007). *Maternal and Neonatal Tetanus.* The Lancet, 370: 1947-1959

6. Michel Odent (2008). *Neonatal Tetanus.* The Lancet, 371/9610. pp 385-386.

7. The National Clinical Training Network (2007). *Pelatihan Asuhan Persalinan Normal Bahan Tambahan Inisiasi Menyusu Dini.* USAID. pp 16 (step 30).

8. Country Profile: Indonesia. JHPIEGO. Retrieved from: www.jhpiego.org/about/cntryprofiles/CPindonesia.htm

9. Jose N. Tolosa, Dong-Hyuk Park, David J. Eve, Stephen K. Klasko, Cesario V. Borlongan, Paul R. Sanberg (March 2010). *Mankind's first natural stem cell transplant.* Journal of Cellular and Molecular Medicine, 14/3. pp 488-495.

10. Robin Lim (Summer 2001). *Lotus Birth: Asking the Next Question.* Midwifery Today, Issue 58. pp 14.

11. Newborn jaundice. MedlinePlus Medical Encyclopedia online. Retrieved from: www.nlm.nih.gov/medlineplus/ency/article/001559.htm

12. Ceriani Cernadas JM, Carroli G, Pellegrini L, Otano L, Ferreira M, Ricci C, Casas O, Giordano D, Lardizabal J. (April 2006). *The effect of timing of cord clamping on neonatal venous hematocrit values and clinical outcome at term: a randomized, controlled trial.* Pediatrics, 117(4): e779-86.

13. Ceriani Cernadas JM, Carroli G, Pellegrini L, Otano L, Ferreira M, Ricci C, Casas O, Giordano D, Lardizabal J. (July 2006). *Randomized Controlled Trial Supports Delayed Cord Clamping for Term Infants.* Lamaze Institute for Normal Birth, Volume 3, Issue 3.

14. Kelly Winder. *Cord Blood – Why Delaying Cord Clamping Benefits Your Baby.* BellyBelly online. Retrieved from: www.bellybelly.com.au/articles/birth/cord-clamping-delaying-cord-clamping

15. Kelly Winder. *Cord Blood – Why Delaying Cord Clamping Benefits Your Baby.* BellyBelly online. Retrieved from: www.bellybelly.com.au/articles/birth/cord-clamping-delaying-cord-clamping

16. Kugelman A, Borenstein-Levin L, Riskin A et al. (May 2007). *Immediate versus*

delayed umbilical cord clamping in premature neonates born < 35 weeks: a prospective, randomized, controlled study. Am J Perinatol, 24(5): 307-15.

17. Hasegawa J, Matsuoka R, Ichizuka K, Sekizawa A, Okai T (March 2006). *Velamentous cord insertion: significance of prenatal detection to predict perinatal complications.* Taiwan J Obstet Gynecol 45 (1): 21-5. PMID 17272203.

18. Nora Benachour, Gilles-Eric Séralini (December 23, 2008). *Glyphosate Formulations Induce Apoptosis and Necrosis in Human Umbilical, Embryonic, and Placental Cells.* American Chemical Society.

19. Jeffrey M. Smith (May 4, 2010). *Genetically Modified Soy Linked to Sterility, Infant Mortality in Hamsters – Consumerism, GMOs, Health & Disease.* The Permaculture Research Institute of Australia.

20. Mother-to-child transmission of HIV: UNAIDS Technical Update (October 1998).

21. Prevention of Mother-to-Child HIV Transmission and Management of HIV Positive Pregnant Women (October 2000). South Africa: Department of Health.

22. Sheldon H. Landesman, M.D., Leslie A. Kalish, D.Sc., David N. Burns, M.D., M.P.H., Howard Minkoff, M.D., Harold E. Fox, M.D., Carmen Zorrilla, M.D., Pat Garcia, M.D., Mary Glenn Fowler, M.D., M.P.H., Lynne Mofenson, M.D., and Ruth Tuomala, M.D. (June 20, 1996). *Obstetrical Factors and the Transmission of Human Immunodeficiency Virus Type 1 from Mother to Child.* Women and Infants Transmission Study, N Engl J Med, 334. pp 1617-1623.

Honoring the Third Stage of Labor: The Birth of the Placenta

1. Dr. Inne Susante, Dr I.B. Asawa and Judith A. Fortney Ph.D. *Maternal Mortality in Bali, Indonesia.*

Lotus Birth

1. Künzel W. (April/May 1982). *Cord clamping at birth - considerations for choosing the right time.* Geburtshilfe Perinatol,186(2). pp 59-64.

Placentophagy: Eating the Placenta

1. London Daily Telegraph (April 13,1995).

2. Mark B. Kristal (February 2, 1980). *Placentophagia: A Biobehavioral Enigma (or De gustibus non disputandum est).*

3. Mark B. Kristal (February 2, 1980). *Placentophagia: A Biobehavioral Enigma (or De gustibus non disputandum est).*

4. Mark B. Kristal (1991). *Enhancement of Opioid-Mediated Analgesia: A Solution to the Enigma of Placentophagia.* Neuroscience & Biobehavioral Reviews 15. pp 425–435.

5. Materia Medica, the Journal of Traditional Chinese Medicine.

6. Mark B. Kristal (February 2, 1980). *Placentophagia: A Biobehavioral Enigma (or De gustibus non disputandum est).*

7. BBC News (May 28, 1998). *UK Entertainment Channel 4 rapped for serving placenta.*

8. Joel Stein (July 03, 2009). *Afterbirth: It's What's For Dinner.* Time Inc. Retrieved from: http://www.time.com/time/health/article/0,8599,1908194,00.html

9. Chip Hilton (2006). *Tom Cruise' Placenta Eating Tips.* Postcards from the pug bus. Retrieved from: http://www.pugbus.net/artman/publish/04182006_placenta.shtml

10. Mark B. Kristal (February 2, 1980). *Placentophagia: A Biobehavioral Enigma (or De gustibus non disputandum est).*

11. Tanzania Jane Goodall, Jamanne Athumani (October 1980). *An Observed Birth in a free-living Chimpanzee (Pan troglodytes schweinfurthii) in Gombe National Park.* Primates, 21(4). pp 545-549.

12. Janneli Miller. *Traditional Chinese Medicine Placenta Preparation.*

Are there Vampires in the Birth Rooms?

1. BMJ. 2011 Nov 15;343:d7157. doi: 10.1136/bmj.d7157

2. Indian Pediatr. 2002 Feb;39(2):130-5

3. Journal of Tropical Pediatrics, Vol 58, No. 6 2012

4. J Perinat Neonat Nurs r Vo 2012. *Rethinking Placental Transfusion and Cord Clamping Issues.* Judith S. Mercer, PhD, CNM, FACNM, Debra A. Erickson-Owens, PhD, CNM

5. http://midwifethinking.com/2011/02/10/cord-blood-collection-confessions-of-a-vampire-midwife/

6. http://midwifethinking.com/2011/02/10/cord-blood-collection-confessions-of-a-vampire-midwife/

7. http://www.whale.to/a/morley17.html

8. http://www.babycenter.de/a36661/warum-ist-nabelschnurbluteinlagerung-umstritten#ixzz3EKUNPq4X

9. http://www.epistemonikos.org/de/documents/e068abb1a37d6f4c343068377945144da56c483f?doc_lang=en

Recommended Films, Reading and Resources

Films

Guerrilla Midwife by Déjà Bernhardt

Tsunami Notebook by Déjà Bernhardt

Orgasmic Birth by Debra Pascali-Bonaro

What Babies Want by Debby Takikawa

The Business of Being Born by Abby Epstein w/Ricki Lake

Birth as We Know It by Elena Tonetti

Music

Monkey God Complex by Hanoman & the Soul Doctors

Books

Lotus Birth A Ritual For Our Times by Women of Spirit and Shivam Rachana

Placenta: the Gift of Life by Cornelia Enning,

Impact of Birthing Practices on Breastfeeding by Mary Kroeger CNM

Yoga untuk kehamilan Sehat, Bahagia & Penuh Makna by Pujiastuti Sindhu

Spiritual Midwifery by Ina May Gaskin

Ina May's Guide to Midwifery by Ina May Gaskin

Prenatal Yoga by Jeannine Parvati Baker

Conscious Conception by Jeannine Parvati & Rico Baker

Artemis Speaks by Nan Koehler

Birth Book by Raven Lang

Blessingway Into Birth: A Rite of Passage by Raven Lang

Gentle Birth Choices by Barbara Harper and Suzanne Arms

Active Birth: The New Approach to Giving Birth Naturally by Janet Balaskas

Immaculate Deception II: Myth, Magic and Birth by Suzanne Arms

The Scientification of Love by Michel Odent

The Farmer and the Obstetrician by Michel Odent

Gentle Birth Gentle Mothering by Dr. Sarah J. Buckely

Choosing Waterbirth by Lakshmi Bertram

Holistic Midwifery Vol 1 & 2 by Anne Frye

Midwifery: Best Practice by Sara Wickham

Birth Models that Work by Robbie Davis-Floyd

The Child Within the Lotus by Margaret Stephenson Meere

Celebrating the Cycle Guiding Your Daughter into Womanhood by Marie Zenack

How to be a Family the Operating Manual by Howard B. Shiffer

The Book of Chakras: Discover the Hidden Forces Within You by Ambika Wauters

Hands of Light by Barbara Ann Brennan

Wheels of Light: Chakras, Auras, and the Healing Energy of the Body by Rosalyn Bruyere

When Things Fall Apart by Pema Chödrön

But a Passage in Wilderness by Margo Berdeshevsky

Beautiful Soon Enough by Margo Berdeshevsky

Essays on Departure: New and Selected Poems 2006 by Marilyn Hacker

Other Books by Robin Lim

After the Baby's Birth, a Complete Guide for Postpartum Women

Eating for Two... Recipes for pregnant and Breastfeeding Women

Obat Asli... The Traditional Healing Herbs of Bali

ASI Eksklusif Dong (in Bahasa Indonesia)

Ibu Alami (in Bahasa Indonesia)

Butterfly People (a novel)

The Geometry of Splitting Souls

Indonesia, Globe Trotter's Series

Are there Vampires in the Birth Rooms?

The Necessary Question of Infants' Human Rights at Birth...

Ibu (mother) Robin Lim, Grandmother and Certified Professional Midwife with the North American Registry of Midwives, Integrated Midwives of the Philippines, and Ikatan Bidan Indonesia, is a founder and an executive director for Yayasan Bumi Sehat (Healthy Mother Earth Foundation), an international not-for-profit organization located in Indonesia. "Lola" (grandmother) Robin, as she is known in the Philippines is a founder and board member for, Wanita dan Harapan (Women and Hope) Philippines, a not-for-profit organization.

Parents, grandparents, aunts, uncles, siblings, families, midwives, doulas, doctors, nurses, hospital administrators and legislators ... we are BirthKeepers. It is our responsibility to ask the next question concerning human rights in childbirth. As BirthKeepers, it is we who are given the sacred responsibility to protect the mothers and our incoming humans, the newborns, at birth and as they grow, for they are the future EarthKeepers. My question now is: "Are we allowing our health providers to rob our babies of their full potential of health, intelligence, immunity and longevity, at birth?"

In Germany, children under the age of 18 are not eligible to donate blood. Blood donations are generally no more than 500 ml, which is 1/10th of the average adult blood volume. Blood donors must weigh at least 50 kg.

Yet, all over the world, in nearly every single medical institution where babies are born, newborns (usually weighing only between 2 and 5 kilograms (4.4 to 11 lbs.) are being denied up to 1/3 of their blood volume. This happens when the umbilical cord is immediately clamped and cut, by the doctor or midwife, just moments after the baby is born.

At the moment of birth, newborn infants have a blood volume of approximately 78 ml/kg, which means about 273 ml, at an average weight of 3.5 kg. This is what the newborn is left with when the umbilical cord is immediately clamped and cut.

Research has shown that when umbilical cord-clamping is delayed for 5 minutes, a newborn's blood volume increases by 61% to 126 ml/kg, for an average total of 441 ml. This placental transfusion amounts to 168 ml for an average 3.5 kg (7.7 lb.) infant. One-quarter of this transfusion occurs in the first 15 seconds, and one-half within 60 seconds of birth.

Is taking 1/3 of a mammal's blood supply harmful? How then can it be legal for hospital protocols and practices to harm newborns, by robbing them at birth of so much of their blood? I have reviewed the extensive research and the evidence, and found absolutely NO benefits for newborn babies, when their umbilical cords are immediately clamped and cut at the time of birth. In fact, the studies prove this to be a harmful practice.

At the time of birth up to 1/3 of each baby's blood supply is traveling from the placenta via the umbilical cord to the baby. Calling this blood "cord blood" is doublespeak, intentionally ambiguous language, meant to fool parents into misunderstanding. The fact is, the blood present in the umbilical cord at the time of birth is the truly the BABY'S blood.

No parent would sign a waiver (often presented in fine print as part of a long informed consent, given to mother when she arrives at a hospital in labor) giving away 1/3 or any amount of the baby's blood. Yet, thousands of times, every day and night, parents are deluded into giving away a significant part of their baby's precious blood supply! The majority of parents in the world are not even asked if the baby's umbilical cord may be immediately severed.

I am quite sure that if I were to remove 1/3 of even one adult patient's blood, without his or her consent, it would be considered a crime. There would be media outcry against me, and I would be prosecuted. How then is it that people tolerate the same unfair treatment of human neonates?

A mountain of research shows that by simply delaying the clamping and cutting of babies' umbilical cords, our newborn children suffer less trauma, fewer inner cranial hemorrhages, and have higher stores of iron at 4 months of age, and even up to 8 months after birth.[123] The nutrients, oxygen and stem cells present in the blood transfused into babies by the placenta, when cord severance is delayed, ensures that the body's tissues and organs are properly vitalized, supplied with energy, and nourished. This translates into improved health, heightened immunity, increased intelligence and potential longevity.

In addition, keeping the umbilical cord intact for some time at birth means that the baby must stay skin to skin with mother. This eliminates or greatly reduces the potential for birth trauma. Research has proven that babies born without trauma enjoy an intact capacity to love and trust. (Michel Odent OBGYN "The Scientification of Love, see entire book)

The simple, natural, common-sense practice of giving the placenta time to do its job, of delivering to the baby his or her full blood supply, has been criticized and NOT implemented by the very doctors and hospitals who have taken an oath, to "Never Do Harm."

The imposed medical habit of immediately clamping and cutting babies' umbilical cords has not been with us so long (just over 200 years) and yet, in the minds of many healthcare providers it is erroneously considered "normal" and "necessary." Clearly the research proves it is not necessary, nor is it evidenced based practice.

> "Another thing very injurious to the child, is the tying and cutting of the navel string too soon; which should always be left till the child has not only repeatedly breathed but till all pulsation in the cord ceases. As otherwise the child is much weaker than it ought to be, a portion of the blood being left in the placenta, which ought to have been in the child." ~ Erasmus Darwin, Zoonomia, 1801

The habitual practice of immediate umbilical cord clamping and cutting began in the 1960s when an unproved hypothesis or theory arose among physicians thinking that immediate cord severance would prevent jaundice. If this is true, why do so many babies who have had their cords immediately clamped and cut need phototherapy for pathological jaundice? Research has proven that there is no greater risk of pathological jaundice for newborns whose cord clamping and cutting is delayed.

Another theory was that early cord clamping would prevent Polycythemia, or too much hemoglobin. Some research does show an increased concentration of hemoglobin in the delayed cord clamping group, but it has not harmed babies, nor is it a significant argument for immediate cord severance. [4]

When immediate umbilical cord clamping and cutting was introduced, it was never questioned. NO research was conducted to determine if it was a safe practice. It was just done for convenience. Doctors, nurses and midwives began to follow the trend, like sheep wearing blinders. Later, they justified it with myths about delayed cord severance causing jaundice. Few asked the questions I am asking today; "What about the Baby?" "What are the Babies' human rights?" "Is the practice and protocol of immediate umbilical cord severance harming our children?" "Is it sabotaging breastfeeding and bonding?" "Is it impairing our children's birthright to their full potential of health and intelligence?" At this junction of herstory and history, many BirthKeepers are asking these very questions. [5]

Research proves that immediate or early umbilical cord severance is detrimental to our newborn children, but no one seems alarmed. Are we hypnotized? Why are we trusting medical professionals, who profits from denying our offspring their very blood? Stealing blood is what vampires do!

Thinking, caring parents and grandparents have concluded that OBGYNs and midwives who insist on routine, immediate umbilical cord cutting are simply protecting their right to practice with impatience, and what they deem 'efficiency,' with no regard for the rights of the baby, who cannot protest.

Another issue is financial profit. Stem cells are valuable, blood is valuable, and hospitals sell babies' blood for transfusions and for research.[6] Many parents are asked to donate their babies cord blood to science or to help others. Did you know umbilical cords are marketed for transplants? Placentas have also been sold to cosmetic companies to be used in beauty supplies, though this is now much less common.

In some countries (especially the US), fear of litigation has been used to justify early cord-cutting. In 1995 the American Academy of Obstetricians and Gynecologists (ACOG) released an Educational Bulletin (#216) recommending immediate cord clamping in order to obtain cord blood for blood gas studies in case of a future lawsuit. They did this because deviations in blood gas values at birth can reflect asphyxia, or lack of. Lack of asphyxia at birth is viewed as proof in a court of law that a baby was healthy at birth.

Following an unpublished letter sent to ACOG by Dr. Morley, ACOG withdrew this Educational Bulletin in the February 2002 issue of Obstetrics and Gynecology, the ACOG journal.[7] This action released them of liability resulting from their previous bulletin #216 of 1995. Parents and all BirthKeepers must ask; WHY, if ACOG has withdrawn its erroneous instruction to doctors, to immediately clamp and cut babies' umbilical cords, is it still universally and dangerously practiced?

Midwives and doctors who propose the healthy process of placental transfusion at birth by delaying umbilical cord clamping and cutting are criticized and charged with the burden of proving that letting nature take her course is safe!

The question of cord blood banking arises. First of all, remember that it is actually baby blood, not cord blood. That said, there are two directions parents are encouraged to choose from: banking their baby's stem-cell-rich blood for donation, presumably to help someone in the future, an altruistic idea; or, banking baby's blood for future personal use, should the child develop a disease perhaps treatable by blood transfusion. The most touted of the presumably treatable diseases is leukemia. The probability that a person in the course of his or her life will ever need a stem cell transplant (whether from umbilical cord blood or bone marrow) has been estimated by the University Hospital in Heidelberg at 0.06% to 0.46%, depending on age. Correspondingly low, the probability that one's own cord blood would be used in a transplant is between 1: 1400 and 1: 200,000.[8] The technology to properly store this baby blood is still not adequate to insure that the blood will be useable in the future. Parents are driven by fear and love for their baby to pay between 1,500 and 2,000 euros or more, for the initial "harvesting" of their baby's blood at birth. Storage programs, for between ten and twenty-five years cost between 90 and 120 euro per year. Parents are asked to gamble that technology will advance enough to make their investment useful, should the worst case scenario for their child's health arise. It must be said out loud and precisely: YOUR BABY NEEDS THAT BLOOD AND STEM CELL INFUSION, WITH ALL ITS BENEFITS, AT THE TIME OF BIRTH, AS NATURE INTENDED IT. With that in mind, there is a third option for parents who are convinced of the need for blood banking: to harvest the baby's blood for collection and storage AFTER delaying the clamping and cutting of baby's umbilical cord, allowing for some of the essential transfusion to take place. immediately after birth.

At Bumi Sehat in Indonesia and the Philippines, we have received nearly 7,000 babies safely into the world, in high-risk, low resource settings. All of these babies enjoyed delayed umbilical cord clamping and cutting. Normally we wait 3 hours before doing anything with babies' umbilical cords, and many parents choose keeping the cord and placenta connected to the baby until the cord naturally dries and falls away, or "Full Lotus Birth." Both of my grandsons enjoyed this non-violent practice.

At Bumi Sehat we have experienced NO ill effects to babies through delaying umbilical cord cutting. A small study was done which compared a sample of 30 babies from Bumi Sehat (greatly delayed cord severance) and 30 babies from a local hospital with immediate cord severance. There was NO increased rate of jaundice in the Bumi Sehat babies, and they enjoyed higher hemoglobin.

Our MotherBabies enjoy a breastfeeding rate of 100% upon discharge from all three of our childbirth centers in Indonesia and the Philippines. We attribute this success of breastfeeding to the bright, enthusiastic way in which babies, born at our birth centers, bond wide-eyed and go directly to the breast to self-attach and feed. Delayed umbilical cord clamping and cutting makes it possible for babies to be bright and energetic. Babies subjected to immediate cord severance suffer from newborn anemia and all of their bonding and breastfeeding activities are impaired.

Severe anemia makes any and all newborn activities, such as gazing, crawling toward the breast, nuzzling, staying awake, latching and suckling, nearly impossible. I sing praises to the determined mothers who manage to bond and breastfeed their infants, in spite of immediate cord severance. Humans are super resilient, but that is no reason to abuse them at birth.

No other mammal, except humans, routinely interferes with bonding and breastfeeding by quickly severing the umbilical cords of their offspring.

No matter if you are rich or poor; educated or not; brown, black, white, red, yellow or of mixed race, Muslim, Christian, Buddhist, Hindu, Pagan, Catholic, Jewish or Agnostic, very young or quite mature, if you go to a medical institution for childbirth, your baby will be robbed of up to 1/3 or 33% of his or her/his natural blood supply.

Just say "NO, I will not allow anyone to abuse my newborn by immediately clamping and cutting my Baby's umbilical cord!"

If you were born in a hospital or clinic, it happened to you. If you plan to give birth in nearly any medical institution on Earth, it will happen to your baby, unless YOU demand time for your baby to receive all of the blood he or she is meant to have.[9] Immediate or early clamping and cutting of babies' umbilical cords is the biggest most widespread, medically sanctioned Human Rights issue on Earth! Together, we can make this a thing of the past. May our babies all be blessed by our patience.

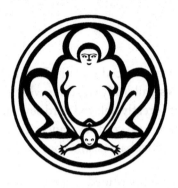

Bumi Sehat Foundation
a not-for-profit organization

Background: Yayasan Bumi Sehat (Healthy Mother Earth Foundation) was founded in Bali in 1995, expanded its services to Aceh immediately after the 2004 tsunami and, in 2010, was an early responder to the earthquake in Haiti. Bumi Sehat is an advocate for marginalized, displaced, low-income people of all faiths and cultures and, from its humble beginnings as an Indonesian not-for-profit organization, has grown to have international impact from its charitable works. In 2013 Bumi Sehat teamed with Wadah Foundation and Direct Relief International in response to the super storm, Haiyan. In the aftermath of the largest typhoon to ever make landfall in recorded history, we have established a medical relief and childbirth camp, in Dulag, Leyte Island, Philippines.

Vision: We believe that access to quality healthcare is a human right. We believe that each individual is an essential societal component of peace and that, by caring for the smallest citizens: the babies at birth, we are building Peace, one Mother, one Child, one Family at a time. Our service is built on three simple principals: Respect for Nature, Respect for Culture, and the wise implementation of the Science of Medicine. Our focus is on culturally appropriate, sustainable family healthcare, gentle maternal health services and optimal infant survival with an emphasis on breastfeeding (the best start and nutritional sustainability for all babies). We believe that each individual is a miracle of hope and a promise of peace.

Activities: In the Village of Nyuh Kuning, Bali, in the village of Gampong Cot, West Aceh, Indonesia, and in Dulag, Leyte, Philippine islands, we operate maternal, infant, family healthcare clinics. Our patients come from all parts of Bali and Aceh and Leyte. They include displaced peoples, homeless, survivors of economic and natural disasters. Wanders/explorers from all over the planet have also found a gentle place to have their babies, with our midwives. Bumi Sehat never turns anyone away, unless it is medically necessary, and in that case, we continue our support. We provide early responder care in the advent of natural catastrophes. Bumi Sehat operates Youth Centers in Bali and in Aceh. We provide programs for the elderly, projects supporting education and capacity building, organic gardening for food security and we work for environmental protection.

Please help Ibu Robin and the Bumi Sehat team
create Peace on Earth, one Precious Baby at a time.
Donations can be made through: www.**bumisehat.org**

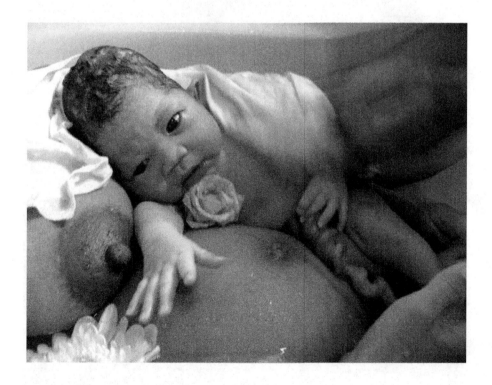

"Imagine a world in which every human is born
with an intact capacity to Love. Now let's create it!"

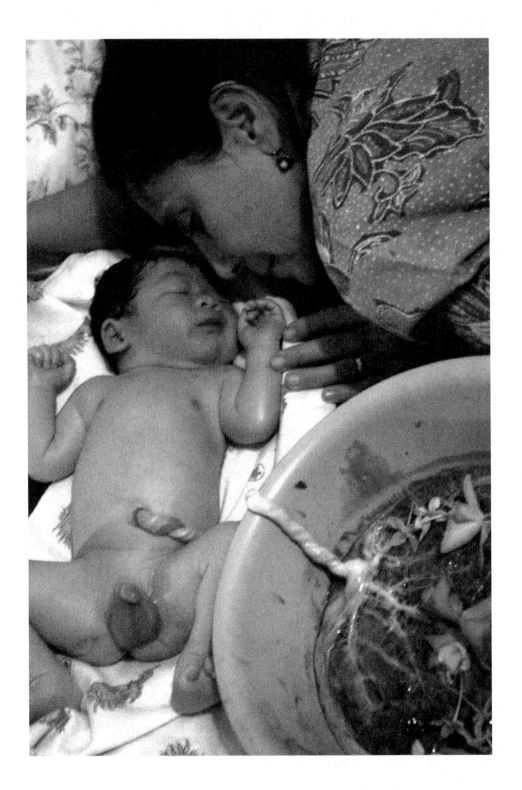

190

About the Author

Ibu (mother) Robin Lim, Grandmother and Certified Professional Midwife with the North American Registry of Midwives, Integrated Midwives of the Philippines, and Ikatan Bidan Indonesia, is a founder and an executive director for Yayasan Bumi Sehat (Healthy Mother Earth Foundation), an international not-for-profit organization located in Indonesia. "Lola" (grandmother) Robin, as she is known in the Philippines is a founder and board member for, Wanita dan Harapan (Women and Hope) Philippines, a not-for-profit organization.

Ibu Robin is also an accomplished author and has been celebrated for her service and charitable works with marginalized people in need. In 1991 she published After The Baby's Birth, the first complete work on the subject of women's health after childbirth. In 2009 Ibu Robin's daughter, Déjà Bernhardt, released an award winning documentary Guerrilla Midwife on the work of her mother, Bumi Sehat and the importance of gentle birth for a peaceful planet. Ibu Robin also wrote the script for the documentary directed by Déjà, Tsunami Notebook.

> *""My inspiration is my family: husband Wil and my eight astounding children: Déjà, Noël, Zhòu, Lakota, Zion, Thoreau, Hanoman & EllyAnna, ages 38 to 8. Three of the most profound moments in my life were receiving my granddaughter Zhouie and grandsons Bodhi & Tashi into my hands, at home. I follow the heartbeat and footsteps of my Filipino Grandmother, Vicenta Munar Lim, a Hilot and traditional birth attendant in the Baguio mountain region of Luzon, Philippine Islands. Before, during and after WWII, she served as a healer and baby catcher for her people. Om Shanti"* ~ Ibu Robin

Awards:

2005: Women of Peace Award by the Women's PeacePower Foundation.

2005: Asian American Volunteer Person of the Year award, shared with her daughter, Déjà Cresencia Jehle Bernhardt.

2006: Alexander Langer International Peace Award.

2011: CNN Hero of the Year

2012: BirthKeeper of the Year, in memory of Jeannine Parvati from the Association of Pre and Peri-natal Psychological Health.

Praise for Placenta the Forgotten Chakra ...

"This lovely and compelling book is an instant classic that belongs in every childbirth library. On this fascinating journey through scientific research, yoga philosophy, folklore, ritual, psychology, midwifery, anthropology, and spirituality, readers will delight in discovering that this ode to placentas is also a guide to the third and fourth stages of labor: the birth of the placenta and the immediate postpartum, a precious time richly bathed in hormones and love that internationally renowned "guerrilla midwife" Robin Lim suggests not simply be severed by cutting the umbilical cord and separating baby from placenta. The significance of the hormone-rich placenta as a chakra, a locus of shared spiritual as well as physical conversion, between mother and baby is profoundly illuminated. With poetic reverence, Robin excavates ancient wisdom while empirically creating, discovering and reinterpreting forgotten practices and rituals involving placentas and umbilical cords with beautifully impressive and lifesaving results. Sound research, clinical observation, and a culturally inclusive worldview that dares to posit love as vital to human health and survival yields detailed instruction in methods and rituals rich in reverence and visionary faith in the human body and spirit to be born into wholeness."

~ **Eden Gabrielle Fromberg, DO, FACOOG, DABHM**
Holistic Obstetrics & Gynecology, New York City

"The evidence overwhelmingly suggests that the "best practice" for maternity care is a holistic, non-invasive model, which is geared to supporting natural processes. Can we afford to postpone mounting an all-out effort (global in scope) to protect mothers, babies, and breastfeeding and to stop the assault on normal, non-invasive childbirth?"

~ **Mary Kroeger, BSN, CNM, MPH**
Impact of Birthing Practices on Breastfeeding
Protecting the Mother and Baby Continuum

ABOUT CHAKRAS... In the many interpretations of the chakra system some include Bindu, and some do not. In my studies and experience, I have come to love the Bindu as the Moon chakra, and so I include it here. There are no 'wrong' variations of teaching concerning the chakras, remember, it is a growing field of knowledge.

Lightning Source UK Ltd.
Milton Keynes UK
UKOW05f1305111117
312479UK00005B/412/P